# Dr. Huls -

# God's Mechanic

## Manipulative Practice of

## W. J. Huls.

**By:**

**Marilynn Griffith-Fargo**

**Rhonda Marinakis**

**Mike Martin**

ISBN-13:   978-1495479069

ISBN-10:   1495479064

# ACKNOWLEDGEMENTS

This is a collaboration of historical information by students, patients, family and friends of Doctor William Jackman Huls. These are a few of the many lives he touched..

Thanks to the many patients of Doc who shared their experiences. Thanks to Joy Burrow for newspaper clippings, Betty's Photo, and research. Cover art courtesy of Don Hersey. Most photographs courtesy of Mike Martin. Historical Photos are from Doc's Office Walls.

While Dr. Huls was a licensed Osteopath, the field of medicine has changed greatly over the years. Dr. A T Still discovered the field of Body Mechanics, and gave it the name of Osteopathy. Dr. Still was an MD before this. He established the training and licensing for Osteopathy. But after his death, the school he founded edged closer and closer to the MD field. Body Mechanics was no longer taught by Osteopathic Schools. If a student today were to become proficient in the A T Stills methods – he would not be able to claim the name nor licensing of Osteopathy. The current Osteopathic training has nothing to do with Dr. Stills discoveries.

So while there are practitioners of Dr. Stills methods all around the country today – there is no "standardized" name for the field.

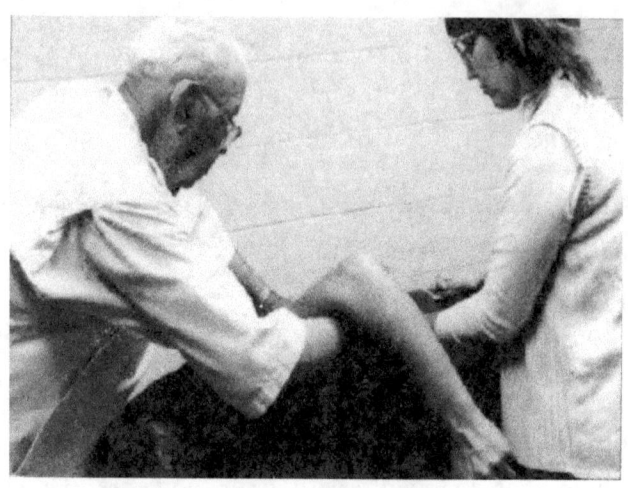

**Marilynn and Doc Huls**

# TABLE OF CONTENTS

# Miracle or Hoax – 1

It hadn't been a good week, or month, or even couple of years for that matter.  In the early years of my marriage – I started having crippling headaches and sinus problems.  After a while, Aspirin wouldn't touch them, and my sinuses started getting more and more congested.  I tried half a dozen or more pain killers, drugs, and decongestants – mostly prescription.  Each day was an eternity – spring allergies added to the fever, pain and infection.   Then the next treatment of choice became driving a stainless steel tube up one nostril and then the other with a wooden mallet to allow flushing out the maxillary sinus cavities.  It was painful, but offered some relief for a few weeks, and then the Doctor would do it again. The black eyes took a while to heal. I spent most of my time resting and trying to recover.  Depression added to the problems.  Day to day life didn't hold much – and luckily my husband was very supportive.

After a few sessions – my Doctor was having trouble finding a new place to drive the tube – everything was so swollen and scarred, the procedure became even more painful.  One day last week he paused before hitting the tube.  He looked at my sinus area, and put down the tube and wooden mallet.  He went to his office, and a few minutes later, returned and told me that this wouldn't work anymore.  He said the only choice was surgery – to remove some of the supportive bone structure with reconstructive surgery. And it could alter my face. That all happens next Tuesday.

I went home in a daze and drug fog, and just went to bed and cried. My husband Bob mentioned that a friend at work had recommended a local Manipulative Osteopath who could work wonders. If it might delay my surgery….

We drove through touristic Scottsdale to Professional Plaza – Suite 7A, W. J. Huls, D.O. The receptionist handed me the usual paperwork. Current complaints? The receptionist gave me another paper to authorize treatment. "Consent to any treatment or OPERATION." Was I trading one surgery for another?"

The receptionist seemed amused at my concern and reaction. She smiled and said "Oh, honey – this is for structural surgery – manipulation – Osteopathic Manipulation." I sat waiting in the reception room – listening to the voices of others. "Doctor did wonders for my grand-daughter. She hasn't had a bit of trouble since." "…. Well, I couldn't even get out of bed without help before." Added another, "He certainly has helped me."

So here I am, sitting on a massage table in a cold dim room – with straps and harnesses hanging on the wall. My stay in the hospital had left me very weak. The mountain of antibiotics and antihistamines I was still taking kept me drugged. I'm trying to decide whether to stay or walk out, when the door opens, and in walks an elderly hunched over man with old glasses, two hearing aids, one good hand (with noticeable nicotine stains) and one stump that included  half a hand and part of a thumb.  I wasn't impressed, actually slightly more depressed.  He looked at my card, then looked up and smiled and said: "Some sinus problems, eh."  I wanted to hit him, and was ready to walk out.  By then, he was behind me, with his hands on either side of my neck – feeling my pulse – running his hand

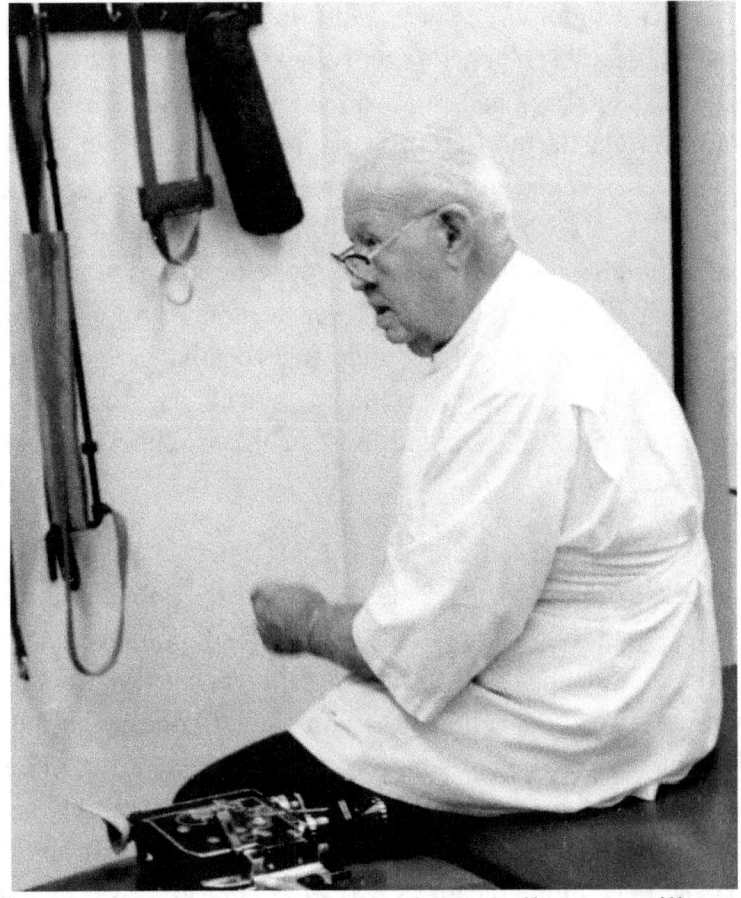

down my spine from the base of my skull to my tailbone. The nurse, Betty, told me to lie on my back.  It took quite a while to make it.  My head stabbed pretty badly. Hesitating occasionally – he ran his hands forward feeling my jaw bone, temples, and forehead. "You don't need surgery, honey," he said, kindly, his eyes shining with inner delight at his discovery.

He walked to the front of the table, and reached into my mouth with his gloved good hand – felt around at the roof of my mouth. Betty said: "It will only pain for an instant, dear." Then his finger began to push steadily. Pain shot through my head in all directions simultaneously! I saw a bright flash of light. Like a miracle – the fluid which had been stopped up in the Eustachian tube receded, like water sipped through a straw. I could hear better immediately, and the pain below my left eye was gone! He turned and walked out of the room without saying a word. I waited for him to return, and after 10 minutes or so, his nurse Betty came in and said I could go. I looked at a mirror on my way out, and most of the swelling I always saw – was gone.

That was too simple. It can't work. I guess I just bought a few more days before surgery. Bob drove me home – and it was quiet in the car. I rested for a few days – and the headache didn't come back. My sinuses were acting normal, and the swelling was completely gone. What just happened? One of our MDs remarked about how wonderful the medications worked to clear out the infection, saving me from surgery. I didn't tell him that I had stopped all medications two weeks before; I was eating normally, and sleeping like a baby. I didn't tell him about seeing Dr. Huls because I knew he wouldn't believe me. It wasn't orthodox. It is not accepted procedure. My curiosity was strong.

I wanted to check into Osteopathy, but my chance came sooner than I thought. Six months after my first treatment with Dr. Huls we were blessed with the birth of a beautiful girl. An alert MD discovered she had a congenital hip dislocation. This is where the head of the bone, called the "femur" is not seated into the hip socket as is normal. Somehow, at a point before, during, or immediately following birth, this positions itself on the lip of the socket. If left uncorrected, the child has a difficult time learning to walk, and has a peculiar lunge to his or her step.

The "accepted procedure" for correcting a congenital hip is a series of castings, designed to help this femur bone to slip back into its correct place. The castings are heavy and unpleasant. Seeing your child like that would be heart wrenching, and sometimes the cost could be hard to meet. Sometimes a few weeks is enough time, others may need several months of castings, teasing the femur into place. We were also informed that there are always a few cases that casting does not help.

We called Dr. Huls' office. We were told that he had a technique for correction through manipulation. So, trusting our instinct, we took our daughter to Scottsdale.

Although Betty had told us that there was no danger, this was, in fact, unorthodox for correcting the condition. We were making a decision which would affect the baby all her life. A mother can understand my feelings as I placed my six week old, precious bundle on the examining table. This was different.... This was not me.... This was much more important, with much higher stakes.

As Dr. Huls examined her, I could feel all of my confidence wane. I wanted to grab her up in my arms and run away! He quietly explained how he was going to correct the dislocation, but his words ran together, my mind whirled. Her very future rested in those gnarled, strong, strange hands.

What appeared to be a simple manipulation left my infant daughter sleeping cozily in my arms a few minutes later. I was sick to my stomach, and the tears began to flow.

Two days later, it was confirmed by a very puzzled Orthopedist. He wouldn't accept the method used, but he sure couldn't find the dislocation which had been there less than a week before. He still wanted to put her in casts.... We refused.

A few years after Dr. Huls worked on my daughter; the proof of his work could be seen in her chubby little legs. She progressed quickly, walking normally at less than one year old. There was never any problem with her running – In fact – to see her today; you would never know that she could have been a cripple all her life.

The technique Dr. Huls used to correct my sinusitis was Osteopathic – yet I have found only a handful of physicians in the world aware of and capable of such manipulation in the cranial region. The technique he used to correct our daughter's hip was also Osteopathic, yet orthopedists – Osteopathic or not, seem to favor the long, expensive, inconsistent system of castings.

I just hung around the office, making mental notes. I watched an elderly man with a cane hobble into a room. Doc walked in and did some adjustments to his legs as they attached to his hips. Then had him sit in a plain wooden chair and told him to stand up. He reached for his cane, and Doc snatched it away. The patient said he couldn't – and Doc told him to try. He stood up without cane or holding on to anything. Doc said: "Mind if I add this to my collection?" and tossed the cane into a corner with half a dozen others. The patient walked out – he didn't shuffle.

Betty named the patient in another room, and Doc looked annoyed. As I walked into the room, I saw Doc turn off both of his hearing aids. The lady was talking about having Doc check this and that. When he walked in – she complained non-stop about her back, her stomach, and a neck pain that he should be sure to check. Doc checked her neck pulse occasionally saying yes, Umn, and eh - and worked on her for about 5 minutes. As Doc left – she said that he fixed every problem she had told him about and commented on how much better she felt. Then, in the hall, he turned the hearing aids back on.

Betty showed him a bag of brownies another patient had dropped by. Doc tried one, frowned, and said: "They are heavy like rocks." Betty scowled and said "We started at 6am – it's Noon, and you haven't stopped for lunch yet. I'm going to eat some - heavy or not. **Go away**."

They were heavy….

I asked Doc if I could take notes for a possible book. He agreed.

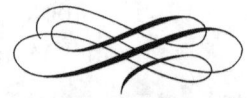

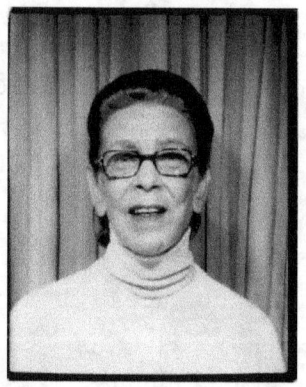

**Betty Bland – Doc's Nurse**

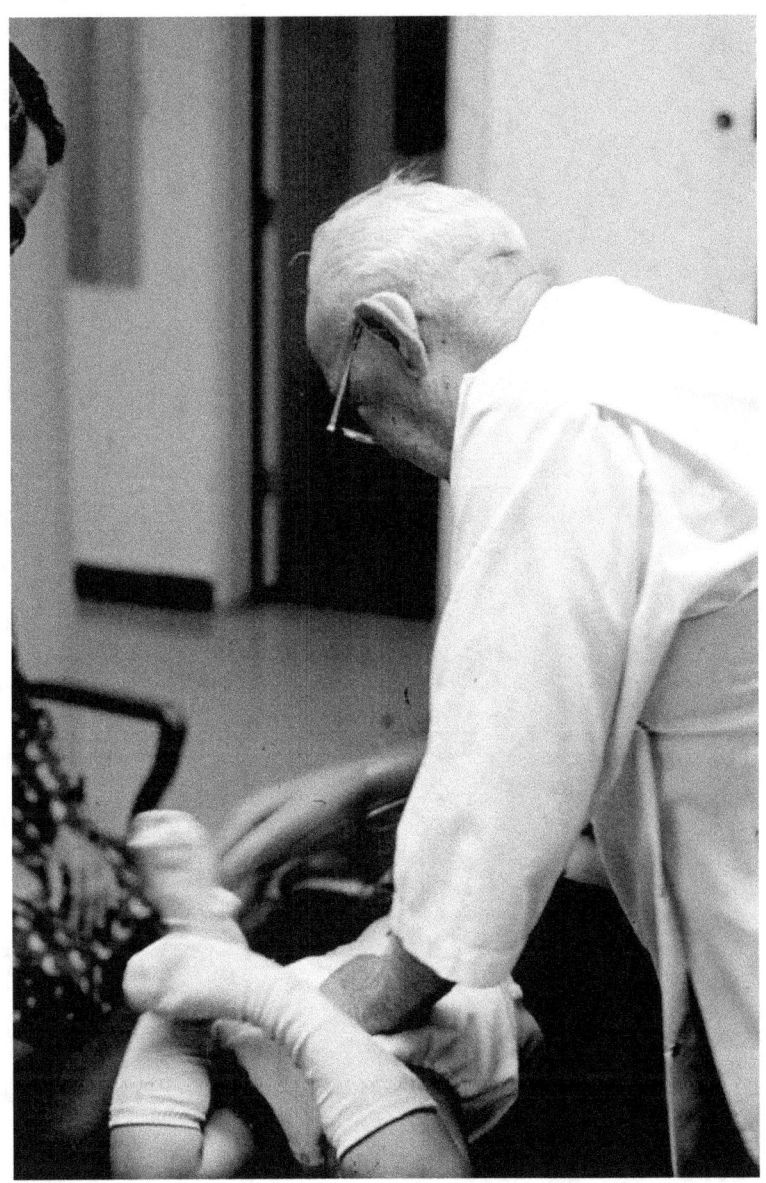

# FIRST ENCOUNTER - 2

"I was born May 9, 1896 in Vernon County, Missouri as William Jackman Huls – although most of my friends and family called me Jackman. I was the only son, and worked the 160 acre ranch near Wolfe, Missouri with my father. We had a fine stock of hogs. It kept us busy, and one day my father came back from town with a sign: "W. T. Huls and Son - Breeders". But this was only to be temporary. My family had decided that I was to become a minister.

One day I was cultivating a field, when the plow and harness attacked, and I was crumpled into a ball trapped between the crown and beam. It took my Father a while to free me, but I couldn't stand and had a terrible shooting pain through my back, down the legs, and up to my head. I passed out while being carried to the house. I told the doctor that my legs were going to sleep.

"I don't doubt that, Jackman," he had answered, closing his black bag and leaving the room, motioning for father to follow. With the preacher, they kneeled and prayed together for understanding and strength. The energy continued to leave my legs, and they became limp and useless. I would probably never walk again.

I hadn't walked for nine months when Father picked me up gently from my bed, saying: "We're heading to Richill, son." I was carried out to the wagon. Mother had the quilts ready, and they settled me in the back of the wagon.

"Son," she said, smoothing my hair away from my eyes, "Father is taking you to a doctor who treated me many years ago." I watched her standing in the yard, waving, as we turned onto the road. The quilts helped cushion the bumps in the road, but it still wasn't a pleasant ride.

Between jolts, I asked my father about this doctor we were going to. "Can he help me to walk again?"

"He cured your mother of headaches back when she was teaching school – before we were married. He has started up a school to teach his "Osteopathy" In Kirksville. But he travels around some, getting to those who need him. I don't understand what he does, but he works different than most. Doctors in town don't hold much chance for you, and we heard that Doc Still can do some pretty wonderful things. Worth a try, right?"

"Sure, father" I said "But what if he can't help?"

Straightening his shoulders, he looked back and met my gaze, "We must trust in the Lord. Life is for living, to the good Lords got work for you, somehow, With or without those legs."

Doctor Still was treating people at the hotel. We waited in the lobby, and soon it was our turn. Father carried me into the room.

"On the table, please," said the elderly man who met us. Curiosity overcame my fear, and I looked at Dr. Still. He didn't look different than other doctors I'd seen. He had grey hair that spilled off his head into a fine mustache and beard, neatly trimmed. One pant leg was tucked neatly into a riding boot, and the other escaped down to the boot top.

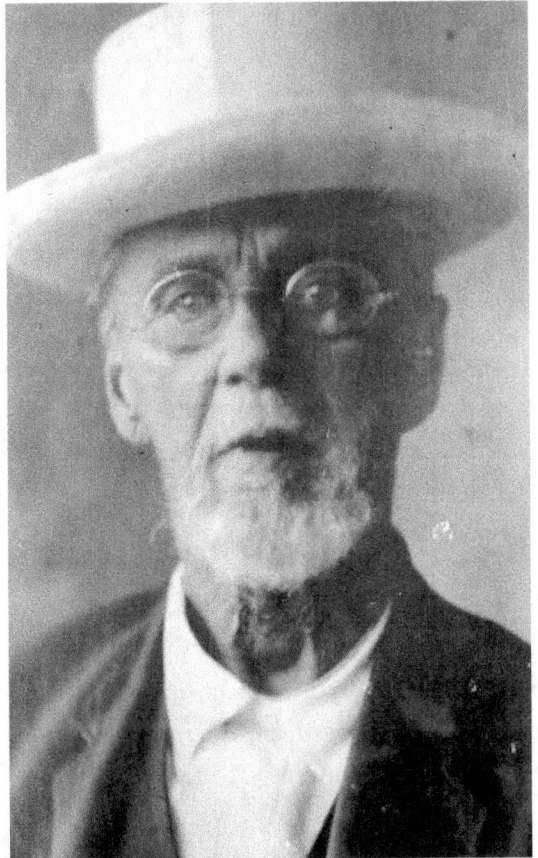

Andrew Taylor Still D.O.

Where's your bag? I asked. "All I need," the doctor answered, amused, "is right here in my hands, son." He motioned for my father to take a seat, and helped me lie down on my stomach. He began to feel my spine - carefully, gently probing. His hands were gentle, confident, and I relaxed a little.

"Doctor Still, "my father began, "He hasn't been able to walk for many months. Not since the accident. Anyways, doctors over in Wolfe say there's nothing to be done…." His voice trailed off….

"Sir," Dr. Still explained, "Doctors have a lot to learn about the human body, even if they don't want to think so. We are machines – God's machines. And we get our belts and framework out of alignment, just like any other machine. Osteopaths are God's Mechanics."

All of this time, his hands had run along the spine. "Here is your trouble." His voice cracked with excitement, and a chill ran through me, as if the very words had been electric!

"This is going to be a little painful boy" he warned, lifting a leg backwards into an uncanny position. Applying body force, he twisted and quickly he was finished. Pain shot through my back as if I were being snapped in two. I yelped, but the pain was already gone. My father leaped to attention – stepping towards the table with concern shadowing his face. Dr. Still massaged my lower back, calmly, as if he hadn't done a thing. Then, standing back, he went about lighting the corn cob pipe he extracted from a vest pocket. Taking a long, purposeful puff, he smiled.

I lay there, almost afraid to breath. It all seemed so strange! I trusted my father, but I have never been handled like that before.

"All right, boy," directed the doctor, "Let's get you off the table and see how you walk." He pulled me around and up into a sitting position – letting my feet dangle over the edge.

"But," I stammered, "I…. I…." I looked at my Father, questioning….

My father stood there, looking perplexed. Then he slowly nodded, looking at the doctor for reassurance. "Son, if the doc says you can…."

My heart was pounding wildly as they helped me stand down, and get my balance. Then they stepped away. I bit my lip and caught my breath. I was almost certain that I could feel my legs beneath me for the first time in nine months. With a new surge of faith, I could begin to feel pins and needles shooting down my legs. I could actually feel my weight on the soles of my feet. Shakily I moved one foot forward… then took another step… and walked!

I had tears and a huge lump in my throat, and a soft sob. Tears came freely, and the room seemed to throb with the emotion.

"Thank God," whispered my father through his tears, "Thank God…"

When I reached my dad, and hugged him, we turned to face Dr. Still. "What can we say?"

"Nothin', except what you have already said. It is God that is the Great Benefactor."

We left the hotel, following some words of advice, and started for home. We sat side by side, on the front seat of the old wagon. It was late when we reached the ranch. I gingerly eased out of the wagon and walked to my mother's waiting arms. That night, during the family Bible time, tears of happiness were shared, prayers of thanks given, and a new vow to do God's will was pledged.

A few years later, my dad's health failed, and he was forced to take a job in town. My early training helped keep the ranch going. I got to visit with Doc McGraw, a veterinarian who visited us on occasion. Doc McGraw said I had a special way with animals, and he suggested I consider veterinary medicine as a future. I liked the idea, and thought it would be better for my back to escape the heavy ranch work.

It would be a change, and I would miss all the wonderful times of home, like the summers, when the garden kept growing so fast that the kitchen table overflowed with baskets waiting to be canned. Sometimes the giant kettles on the stove were not enough, and mother and the girls would build fires outside, with the mouthwatering aromas floating around like invisible clouds.

I would miss fall, when the leaves always lost their valiant battle to the nips of frost. Miss the togetherness of father and son, working side by side filling the smokehouse with bacon, hams, and beef. And storing feed for the stock.

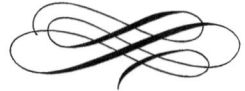

# STUDENT YEARS - 3

I decided to attend Kansas City Veterinary College. Doc McGraw had helped me study for the entrance exam. I was the youngest in a class of 146 students. I took a second floor room about 8 blocks from my classes. I located a job washing dishes at a restaurant on Truest and 12th Street that paid $2 a week. After rent, I had fifty cents left over.

The studies were rough – Latin, anatomy histology, physiology, and lots of lab work. Many students dropped out that first year, but I made it. I went home for the summer, but was glad to get back to Kansas City in the fall.

I worked at the restaurant again – opening for business – but between the few customers, I got to study. Then I went to school and back to the restaurant again each night. I had Saturdays off, so I got a job selling shoes. During that 2nd year I was asked to assist some of the teachers. That was great because I could learn more, and make some extra money.

One of my instructors said: "Animals can't tell you where they are ailing. Remember to use the blood as your basis for diagnosis. I'm trying to teach you the normal blood picture – then when you do a slide, check for abnormality. Don't listen to people," he warned with a smile, "sometimes it makes a decision a darn sight more complicated." "Remember, people can be mistaken, but the blood, the River of Life, never lies. You don't need a lot of stains and dyes, not if you manage to learn the pure blood picture. Everything is there to see, if you know what to look for. You're learning that here, Jackman, and you're learning it well. Use it in your practice."

During this time, 1915, we were allowed to help at the clinic. One week a middle aged man came into the barn. I asked if he needed help, but he just wanted to look around. He came back every day for a while, and toured the barn while I explained the conditions, the treatments, and pointed out the progress. We became friends, and talked about news, medicine, and treatments.

On my last day in the school year, he mentioned that he knew I was leaving after that day for a few months. He said: "I'm leaving town soon, and want to thank you for being so nice to me – showing me around and all."

"Veterinary medicine really is a wonderful helpmate for human practice – as Animals and Humans have much in common. There is a great similarity in the blood and even in pharmaceutical dosages. I drop in whenever I'm in town to see what new has been developed in the way of research. Besides," he added with a wink, "I meet some nice folk that way."

"You'll make a good vet," he prophesized, "and you'd make a darned good medical doctor too, if you ever decided to. If you ever get up to Rochester, in Minnesota, please come to see me. My brother and I have a medical clinic there. "And," he emphasized, "if you ever need any help, just let me know."

I thanked him, but had to ask: "Who do I ask for? Who are you?"

"Mayo's the name," he answered, taking my hand in a parting gesture, "Charles Mayo..." With that he turned heel and disappeared around the corner of the barn.

The third year of school flashed by, and then the next week – Graduation. I was happy, but discovered there was a twenty-five dollar graduation fee – and I didn't have it. I was crushed and prayed deeply, asking God to give me a reason for this strange twist. I couldn't argue God's Plan, but I didn't know where to turn.

The head of the College, Dean Stewart, learned of my predicament and called me to the office. He placed twenty five dollars on the desk in front of me. I stammered "Thank you. I'll pay you back every penny...." And I did.

A few weeks later, I began my own practice in Douglas, Kansas. I couldn't afford a regular office, but the folks at the drugstore let me use their place. And the girls at the telephone office next door took my calls. I didn't have any problem becoming known – in my first week, I diagnosed Anthrax from a blood slide, and saved the whole county from an epidemic.

Shortly after I established the practice, the War broke out, so I enlisted in the Army in 1917. The nicest thing to happen in those years was to meet Olive, and marry her in 1919 while I was still in the service. When I was discharged, we decided to move to Wichita and set up a practice. People learned that I could return barren cattle to production, and that set my reputation. I did quite a bit of traveling, consulting in other areas.

Married life with Olive was wonderful. We gave birth to our first child, Ursula.

The next year, we had a chance to take over a practice in North-Central Missouri. Kirksville was surrounded by good farm land and heavy woods. The town square was the site of a teachers college which had burned down in 1872. Shops and businesses lined the perimeter. The residential area was guarded by giant elms, oaks and maples – a fine place for the family.

While sightseeing one day, I came to a clump of buildings. Many people were scurrying around with books. The sign read:

## AMERICAN SCHOOL OF OSTEOPATHY

### Andrew Taylor Still, founder, 1892

My mind snapped back to that hotel room in Richill. Wonderful, and a bit strange, how things worked out. Then, tipping a mental hat to my benefactor's campus, I continued across the tracks to the location of the new Office.

The office occupied the whole first floor of the building, and there was plenty of room for expansion. There was room to continue my side business of breeding and selling English Setters and Pointers – like I had done in Wichita. Dr. Michael Lane, Pathologist for the area, and a teacher at the Osteopathic School occupied the floor above my new office. One day in February of 1922, he died suddenly while teaching a class. A short time later, the President of the school, Dr. George A Still, nephew of the founder, sent for me.

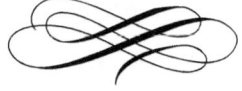

# A TURN IN THE ROAD - 4

"Morning" I said, taking a seat near the large desk. Dr. George Still watched me for a minute, and then blurted out "Why in hell aren't you an Osteopath?"

"I'm a Vet," I stammered, after such an abrupt beginning. Then I added, "And I don't know that I believe in your profession."

"That's a damn poor excuse!" Then, with a grin he said: "Well I still want you to take Dr. Lane's place, teaching Pathology."

I asked: "What makes you think I can teach it?"

Thrusting letters across the broad desk, Dr. Still continued, "These are from Kansas City, from some of the finest pathology men in the country. They say you're qualified. And that's good enough for me." He continued: "I'll pay you a salary, plus tuition-free Osteopathic training.

I asked: "How much without the schooling? I'm not interested in your line of work."

"No deal!" he answered firmly. "I won't have you around here if you won't take the whole package. You'll make a damn good Osteopath if you give it a chance," he added with a wink.

"I can't give you an answer right off.  I'd like to think it over."

"Sure, sure, talk it over with the Missus.  Let me know in an hour or so."  As I left, Dr. Still added: "By the way, we'll give you two and a half years credit on your vet training, and you might as well keep your vet practice going, at least for a while, to help on expenses."

I headed for home and talked it over with Olive. Although the future as an Osteopath held little appeal, the idea of added income was a good one, especially with another child on the way.  I returned to the school and accepted the position.

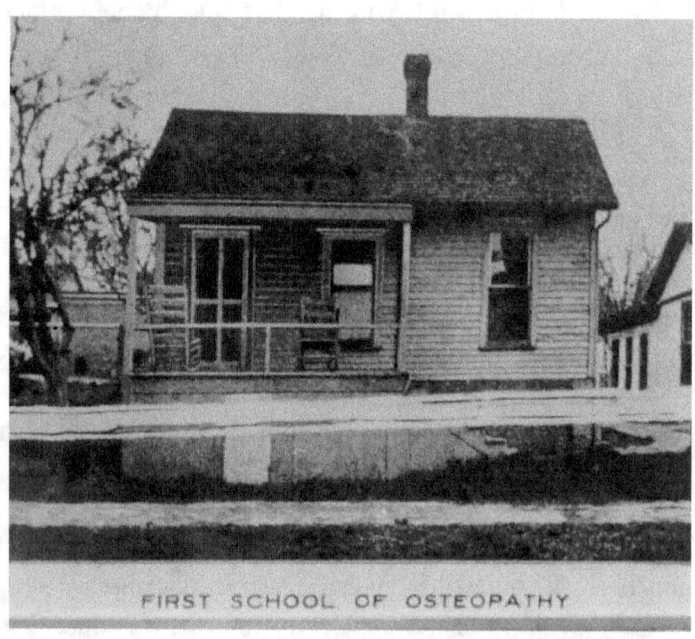

FIRST SCHOOL OF OSTEOPATHY

A few days later, Dr. Roscoe Lyda, who had come from Seattle to care for his ailing mother, and was the most popular Osteopath in town, stopped by my office.

"Good morning, Doctor Huls," he said, offering a hand.

"Coming for your dogs today? " I asked – returning the handshake.

"No, not today, I wanted to talk to you about something else." His eyes sparkled like crystals. "I heard you're going to teach at the college."

"You heard right," I confirmed, "going to start this fall. Have to take the course too. That's part of the bargain. Don't know what a vet will do with Osteopathy, but it can't hurt any I guess." "Dr. Lyda, I've never closed my eyes to any new knowledge. While I'm teaching, I'll be learning. Only time will tell if Osteopathy has anything to offer me. I'm not sold on it yet."

"Pop Still told me to keep my eyes open for the likes of you..." he said, "Special, sensitive, open-minded men make the best technicians, he used to say." Then he offered, "I've got a small class starting soon, teaching Dr. Still's techniques and theories. I want you to join us. I want to teach you true Osteopathy, using just your hands, before that place," he said, nodding towards the school, "has a chance to ruin you."

"Well," I answered, "I appreciate the offer, but I can't afford..."

"Who said anything about charges," he interrupted, I just want you to come. You always strive for the best in your practice here, so just come and watch. Or," he challenged, "Are you afraid you might learn something?"

"I can't turn that down!" I said, "But I can only come when my other work will allow, alright?"

"Good! It's a deal," Dr. Lyda beamed, shook his hand again, and left.

I thought "I guess I owe that much to the man who made it possible for me to even be standing here today!

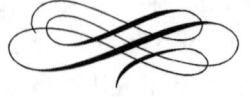

# Searching and Seeking - 5

Everyone was saddened when, in November, Dr. George Still died of an accidental gunshot wound. Dr. George Laughlin, son-in-law of A. T. Still, had been directing the Kirksville College of Osteopathy and Surgery at this time. They had shared classrooms and facilities, but not theory, with the school being directed by George Still. Dr. Laughlin took over both, combining them, using his teaching practices, yet calling it the **AMERICAN SCHOOL OF OSTEOPATHY.** The school had been

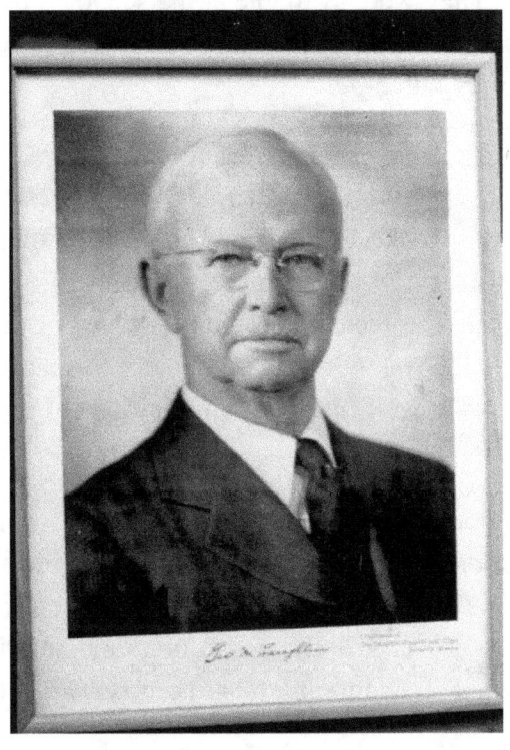

founded by the Doctor who invented Manipulative Osteopathy – A.T Still. But when Cousin George Still had taken over – the school and Osteopathy had taken a giant step away from Manipulative towards a more MD – like style of medicine with surgery and drugs.

Dr. Laughlin took yet another giant step away from Manipulative Osteopathy. As it turns out, the casual deal with Dr. Lyda – the only true link back to A. T. Still would be most important in my life.

Dr. Lyda had begun his classes by having each of the eight students, mostly seniors from the College; purchase a copy of Dr. Still's text book, "Research and Practice." They were available at the school, although they had gathered dust since they were not part of the teaching curriculum by this time.

Twice a week Dr. Lyda demonstrated a point of technique based on the principle, "Structure on tension moves at the weakest point". Then each of them, having wooed into service a suitable test person, practiced that technique until perfected. I selected a Negro by the name of Jack Cole. He was not an easy subject to manipulate, for his body was well-muscled and strong from years of hauling coal.

I soon found that the classes were not enough. They were merely wetting my appetite, so I began visiting Dr. Lyda's office whenever I could. In the office I would observe Dr. Lyda's daily procedure, and application of techniques. The examining table he used was a key to his successful treatment, he explained, designed and manufactured by a blind doctor named Macklin. It differed from any I had ever seen. In place of an immobile flat surface, it had divisions in it to aid in positioning the body for the greatest amount of ease for manipulation. Both ends could be adjusted for proper tilt for the head and upper torso, while the sides could be positioned vertically for use in the lumbar and pelvic regions.

Dr. Lyda worked quickly, confidently. He paid little attention to the patients' own descriptions of their aches and pains, but went right to the cause, which he located in his initial examination.

One day, when I was visiting, Dr. Lyda asked for a treatment. He had never allowed a student to manipulate his cervical region, but I located the cause, and snapped his neck. Dr. Lyda leaped off the table and turned to face me. Then Dr. Lyda spoke, "Although I did not intend for you to actually treat my neck," he scolded, "your treatment was justified and correct." "So," he added, taking his place on the table, "you may continue, please."

A few weeks later, when the classes were finished, Dr. Lyda told us he would be returning to Seattle to continue his practice, but he wanted to pay tribute to the student he felt had gained the most from the course. It was Jack Cole's 'bone-rattler.'

That's what Osteopathy seemed to be. A Good way to make a living, Giving people what they wanted - - a good bone-rattling! It seemed to make them feel better, the principles were sound and moral, but it was only an art. Something he had learned, just like veterinarian medicine. Know your subject, give the patient – human or animal – what he needed, and that was all there was to that. I continued with my Vet practice, teaching pathology, and learning what I could from my courses at A. S. O. It was a busy, happy time, now blessed by the birth of a son, Wilbur.

It was January of 1927, several months before his graduation, when dysentery struck Kirksville. It was the wicked, life-draining type, striking mostly children, and there seemed little to combat it.

"Letitia has taken the dysentery!" Olive blurted out as I came home. "She is so little…!" Her eyes filled with tears, thinking of all the children who had died recently. I called the pediatrician at the College, but he offered no help. Some made it, others didn't he confessed sadly. He recommended the M.D., but even when he came, there was little hope or comfort.

For three days she gradually became worse, soon too weak to eat, and the diarrhea so severe she began to pass blood. Together we prayed for help. Then I remembered something. "Olive, fetch that Dr. Still's book. There's a treatment in there for Dysentery. It's worth a try."

Olive shuddered as I took my six year old daughter into my arms and laid her on the table. Her breath was shallow and raspy, like a dying cat… Her eyes, once bright and alert, were sunken in – dark and unseeing. Her baby soft skin was parched and stretched tightly from one tiny bone to another.

Carefully, with great concentration, I began the treatment as Olive read to me. When we finished, we wept. Our precious Letitia, after so many hours of agony, dozed lightly. She awoke in about fifteen minutes, and I treated her again. I could feel the fever leaving her spine and her body began to respond with a warm perspiration. She slept for four hours and woke up hungry. Olive fed her as the book advised, and recovery came quickly, and soon she was her bubbly, cherub self.

The experience changed me more than it changed my daughter. Osteopathy was no longer an art. Osteopathy - Dr. Andrew Taylor Still's Osteopathy saved my daughter's life when everyone else had said nothing could. To me, Osteopathy came alive as an invaluable Science, and 'Research and Practice' became my medical Bible. I spent hours reading and studying each word and phrase – perfecting my understanding of it.

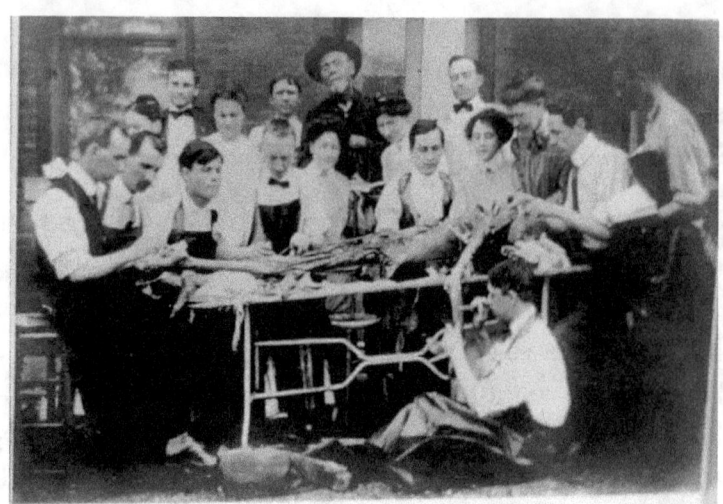

I obtained a cadaver at the College, and each evening, when I had closed my office doors, I went to the College and worked. The dissection I had done in Vet School had been interesting and informative. The work as a teacher of Pathology had been well worth its while. But

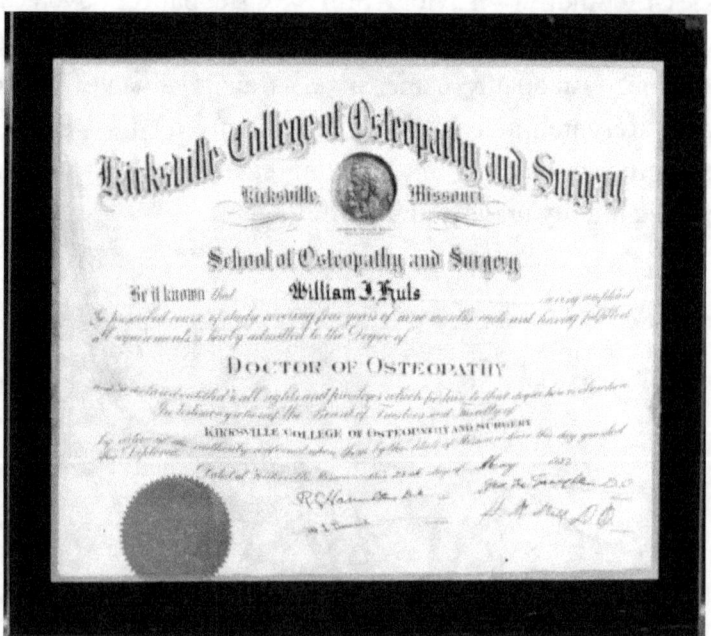

this was different. I was spurred on by the memory of my child, and as Dr. A.T. Still had done after his own child's recovery, I set about learning and proving the theories of anatomical placement so he could truly help others who were in need. When I graduated, I resigned as Pathologist and turned my vet practice over to another, and took an office off the lobby of the Stephanson Hotel. This new practice, much of which I inherited from Dr. Lyda, grew larger and larger.

I didn't solicit any followers, but as Dr. Lyda had done with me, sought out and accepted only those students who were open-minded, sensitive, and sympathetic to Dr. Still's theories.

This turn in the road, going from a Veterinarian to Osteopath, was not any easy one to maneuver. My hunger was for more and more knowledge and it kept me busy most of the time. Olive helped as best she could – as receptionist and book keeper. I wasn't fully satisfied with Dr. Lyda's teachings, and strived to fill in the spaces where the techniques seemed to be lacking. I wanted to explore and enlarge on Dr. Still's findings.

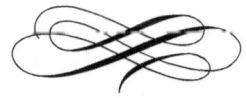

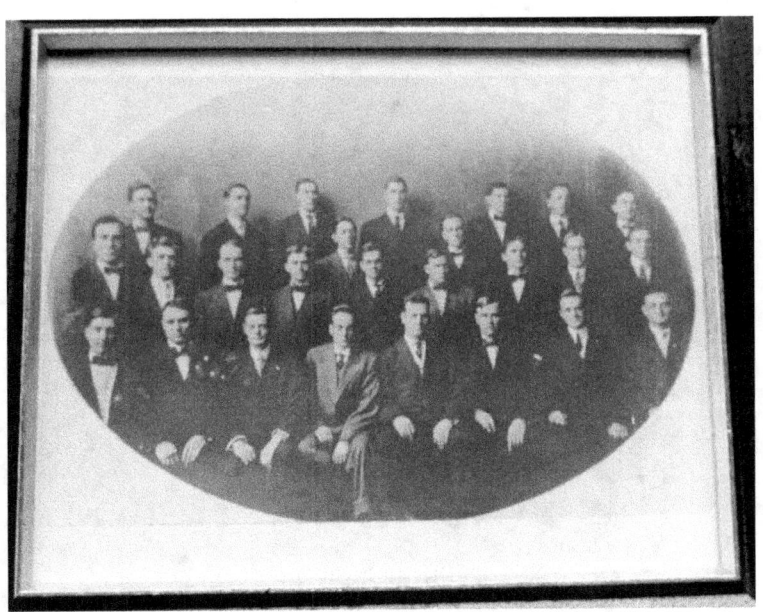

# A SHIFT IN CAREER - 6

There were many at the American School of Osteopathy who did not understand nor accept Doctor Lyda's techniques, and so didn't approve of me. But Dr. Laughlin, who was the head of the school since Dr. George Still's passing, was more open-minded and seemed to enjoy my enthusiasm. Dr. Laughlin spent a great deal of time in Europe, studying with some fine, devoted surgeons and physicians, and shared these techniques with those who were interested. I spent many hours discussing, researching and developing surgical techniques under his tutorship.

One of the most interesting to me was the specific treatment for correcting a fairly common condition, 'unilateral hip displacement', or 'congenital hip'. This condition, Dr. Laughlin explained, had first been diagnosed by a French surgeon, Dupuytren, but until 1886, had been considered impossible to correct. Then a Bavarian surgeon, Hoffa, fathered a method of correction by surgery. Opening the hip from behind and enlarging the socket for the head of the femur. Ironically, the irritating effects of the antiseptics used for such surgeries later led Dr. Lorenz of Vienna, into transferring his energies into a new field called "bloodless surgery." He perfected a technique for manipulation to correct the condition and many others. My studies had led to a complete understanding and knowledge of normal skeletal, muscle, and ligament articulation, so I had a head start in mastering these techniques.

In 1910 I took a few days off, and traveled to Rochester, Minnesota to the Mayo Clinic. Dr. Charlie greeted me, and gave a tour of their impressive facilities. Once he found that I was licensed as an Osteopath, he suggested that I take some additional training with them. I was honored to accept. He sent me to Samantha, Kansas to meet and study with Dr. Murdock, a surgeon.

I was amazed at the way Dr. Murdock could diagnose abnormal conditions. Merely using his hands, for example, he could feel whether an appendix needed immediate surgery or an ice-pack would suffice. I asked him how this was possible.

"Well," Dr. Murdock explained, "you must have your eyes in your fingertips." Placing a piece of glass on the table, he plucked a hair from his head and laid it on the glass. Then he covered this with a tissue. "Find the hair, Dr. Huls," he challenged. Running my fingers over the tissue – I felt nothing. Dr. Murdock followed, hesitated, and then grasping the tissue, turned it over to reveal the trapped strand!

I practiced whenever time permitted, and after about two weeks, the fleshy part of the first finger began to perceive the infinitesimal ridge. I returned to show Dr. Murdock. We worked together to apply the new found sensitivity to locating abnormal conditions of all kinds throughout the body.

Dr. Charles Mayo was pleased with my occasional visits. One day, after describing and demonstrating this "newly-developed skill", Dr. Mayo suggested that not only was this a good tool in diagnosis, but I should try to free restricted organs, lance ovarian cysts, and correct displaced ligaments by this same method – thus eliminating the need for the surgical knife. In truth, many years before, I had begun to use a "bloodless technique" to break cysts in barren cattle, restoring them to production. I continued to practice and expand the use of this technique whenever the opportunity presented itself.

Dr. Mayo also referred me to Dr. Hugh Miller, a brain surgeon at the clinic. I traveled back and forth to these teachers for many years, whenever my own practice would permit. Dr. Miller assured me that I was well-knowledged enough to enter the field of brain surgery, but I declined. I found that type of work too depressing – with a fatality rate at 90%. I wished for better results than that.

By now, the depression years were upon us, and Kirksville was feeling the toll. I moved my practice to Davenport, Iowa in 1937. It took about six months to get settled and send for Olive and the children, but the financial situation did improve. After a few minor moves about town, we took up residence in a large, several story house on 15th and Farnum. It covered about nine lots. There was a separate building, once used as a servant's quarters, and I made this into a kennel. Now I had a place to breed and sell my Irish and English Setters and Pointers, which were in demand all over the country.

In the main house, there were two living rooms, a dining room, kitchen, library, and a solarium – which I used for a hospital. All of this was on the ground floor. Below was a basement, and above were several rooms for the family.

And I invested in a 310 acre farm about 19 miles out of town in 1940, and had two families caring for it. They bred and sold saddle horses, short horn cattle, and Canadian Yorkshire hogs. I liked to go out on the week-ends and help with the chores. It gave me a break from the tensions of the medical practice, and fed my farm-boy tendencies. Letitia and Ursula went away to the University of Iowa, and Wilbur entered the Osteopathic School in Des Moines.

Life was good, and the practice was very successful. Orthodox surgery became obsolete for me, and I discontinued using a knife completely in 1942, referring rare cases to surgeons.

There was one point in my studies which continued to bother me. My studies with Dr. Miller had not given me any techniques for releasing pressure off the brain – returning to natural function. I thought that there should be ways to work with the head – short of the dangerous surgical techniques. I believe that the body holds all the keys for good health – so this area was of concern to me. In the early 40's, I traveled to St. Peter, Minnesota to look up Dr. William Garner Sutherland, an Osteopath who specialized in cranial work. My use of the sensitivity of the fingers was not new to Dr. Sutherland. He taught his students:

"...The fingers should be like detectives, skillful in the art of locating things hidden. His fingers should be able to cipher the sensation signal code found in all the tissues along the backbone cable. The 'finger-feel', 'finger thought' and the 'finger-sight' is the way to read the diagnostic message. The fingers should tarry, firmly, yet gently, yet deeply, on articulation, on ligaments, on muscles here and there, telling the fingers many important things. The fingers should not only feel while diagnosing, but also while treating. Osteopathic technique is governed by and through the intelligent application of the intelligent sense of touch..."

His basis for such technique laid in knowing true structure and anatomy, for without this, he insisted, the sensitivity was useless and even dangerous. And he, himself, refused to pass on certain techniques to those he felt were not qualified. My time was well spent, but I soon had to return to Davenport. I took with me the seeds of the techniques I needed to develop my own techniques in cranial manipulation. Dr. Sutherland's methods were not consistently beneficial in relieving the problem.

I was obsessed with solving this puzzle. I obtained an articulated skull, with each plate hinged, and every evening after office hours, I retired to my room to ponder this mystery. These were the war years of 1942 and 1943, and I was seeing 100 patients a day. Olive became concerned that I was under too much strain – but solving this mystery was important.

One night, in my darkened room, I sat holding the skull while moving my fingertips over each suture, pressing, seeking the key-stone. Suddenly, the skull fell open like a lotus blossom! I wondered if I had just been clumsy, so I re-assembled it, and tried it again. Once more, the skull fell open. Now I concentrated on finding more pressure points, and time and time again, I was successful. I laid my head down on my arms, and went to sleep – too exhausted to show emotion…

The very next morning, an Elder from the Mennonite Community near Davenport came in with his wife and son. The boy, seven years old, was a vegetable. A distorted head bobbled helplessly on the weak shoulders. His eyes, though bright, were unable to focus, and wandered continuously from side to side. Laying him on the table, the bearded father explained that the boy had suffered a birth injury, had never developed, could not speak, and couldn't even turn over by himself. Doctors had told them there was nothing that could be done, but they had come to me in the hopes that I might have an answer.

In my examination, I payed particular attention to the head. I could feel the abnormal condition of the skull, the overlapping of the frontal and parietal. I left the room and returned with the articulated skull. I showed them what I had discovered just last night. I explained to them what I had found on their son, and showed how I thought I could release the pressure. This would allow the cells in that part of the brain to be activated. I told them that I had no way of knowing how much success we would have. After many years of correcting other restrictions, I have seen Nature restore many to health. God willing, this boy would respond the same way.

I watched as the couple discussed their decision in German. After a bit, the father nodded to me, and said: "We want you to try. You have been honest with us, and we trust the Lord will guide you."

After some preparation, I began. Unaware of my surroundings, I concentrated and searched until I located the key points I had found on the skull the night before. I applied gentle yet firm pressure – and felt the bones shift… Ever so slightly… Quickly, I moved to the next point of contact, and again applied steady pressure. I felt the movement. I reminded the couple that I had only removed the blocks, and Nature would do the rest. I didn't know how long it would take, or even what path of action it would follow. They would have to wait and see. About one month later, the little boy <u>Walked</u> into my office….

Soon the Mennonites were bringing their children and families. I treated 700 babies over the next few years. They had been plagued by a birth injury rate of nearly 15%, but with treatments given at two weeks of age, that all dissipated, and the children grew up healthy and normal. The last piece had been added to my puzzle, and my total faith in God and Osteopathy was complete.

As the years rolled past, I continued to use all the knowledge I had obtained. Drs. Mayo, Murdock, Miller, and Sutherland had shared knowledge and techniques with me – and I was able to expand on them. But the very foundation of this success lay in the hands of one man, Dr. Andrew Taylor Still, and his Child of God, Osteopathy. Never would the pressures of Society change his method of practice. God had created man perfect, as a well-balanced machine, and as long as I had my two hands – I would continue to be one of God's Mechanics.

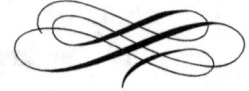

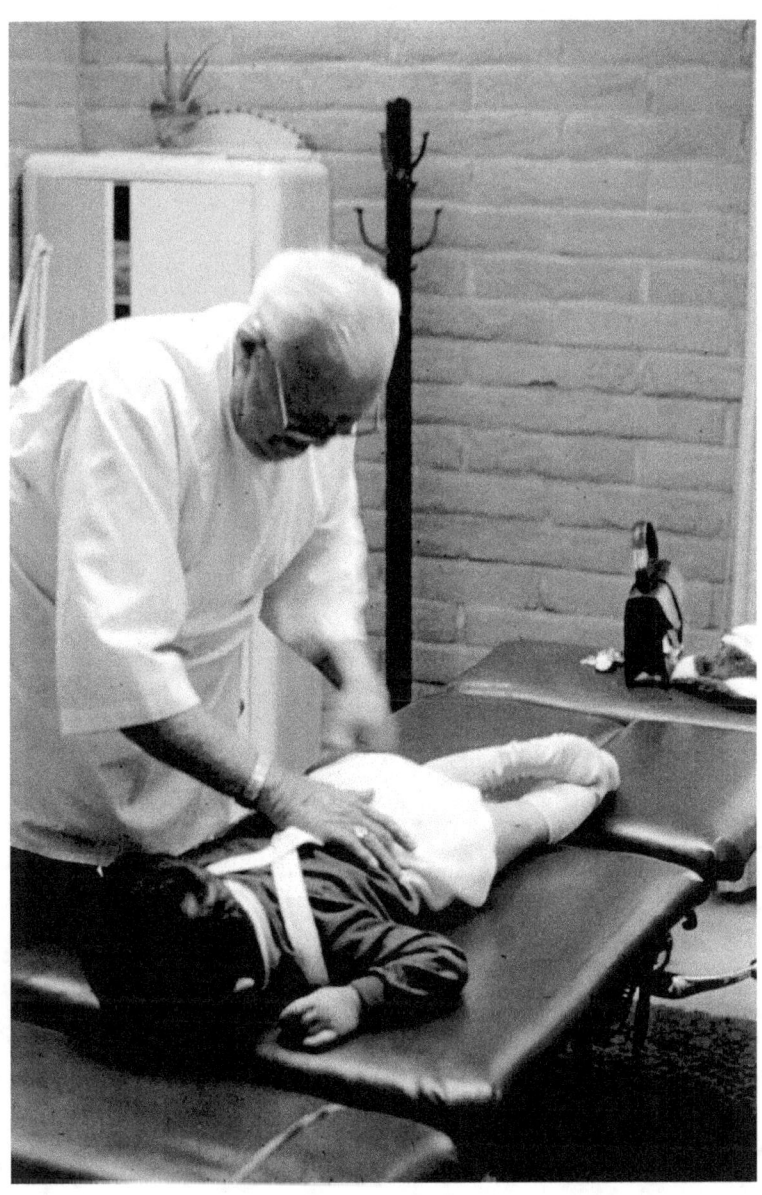

# GOD'S WILL BE DONE. . . - 7

When he graduated from Osteopathic College, my son Wilbur joined me in practice. By this time, my techniques set me aside from other Osteopaths. I had laid down my scalpel, for I had no need for it. Dysfunctions of organs were proven to be caused by restrictions, and when bloodless manipulation removed that cause, the normal motion was restored and surgery was averted. The correction of skeletal displacements relieved the chronic aches, pains, and lack of motion. Other than setting occasional broken bones, orthopedic surgeries were also eliminated.

Olive succumbed to cancer in 1952, and I dove into my practice even deeper to fill the void. In 1953, I married a former patient and friend, Regina Bisch, and again had a helpmate. I spent much of my time away from the office – out on the farm, which was beginning to show the fruits of hard labor. The stock was recognized across the country ad being of a good line, and I traveled around the country selling and buying.

All of the feed was raised right on the farm itself, and whenever harvest time rolled around, I was there to help with the extra work. One day, while running the corn picker, something jammed the blades. Leaving the machine running, I got down and went around seeing what was the problem. I poked at the blades, trying to free them. Suddenly, they freed and instantly, swallowed my gloved hand!

It all happened so quickly, there wasn't even time for pain. I stared blankly at the bleeding mass that just a moment ago had been my right hand. I clutched the wrist to stop the blood flow and looked around for help. I was a great distance from the house, and there was no one in sight. I began a long walk across the field, praying that I could make it before I became too weak.

I only spent a week in the hospital. Wilbur corrected the shoulder which had been dislocated in the accident. Regina and I went to our newly acquired home in Boulder, Colorado so I could mend. When the initial pain subsided, the stump, which only held the thumb, slowly became numb of feeling, except to the sensation of cold, which made it ache.

I had always sworn that as long as I had my hands, I would continue to serve mankind. Now one of them had been taken away. A test, I guess, of my faith and dedication? No – it would not change my pledge. Nearly a year passed before we returned to Davenport.

My son Wilbur had kept my practice while I was gone, and when I returned, Wilbur moved to Blue Grass, Iowa to set up his own practice. I learned to write with my left hand, and to diagnose with the fingertips of that hand. Other than that, there was little change in my technique. I devised intricate maneuvers using straps and belts for added leverage. I continued to use True Osteopathy with all I had added to it.

In April of 1959, Regina and I were on the way to visit relatives in California, and made a brief stop in Arizona. After a day or so in Tucson, I noticed that my hand felt better – the aching from cold was missing. I decided to move to Arizona. Returning to Davenport, I quickly made the arrangements, and became licensed in the state. We moved to Phoenix in May.

We started in Sunnyslope with an office on 19$^{th}$ Avenue and Indian School Road, right near the Osteopathic Hospital. But a few months later – I experienced my first Phoenix Summer, and moved to a home with better cooling in Paradise Valley. I moved the office to North Main Street in Scottsdale – on the Northeast side of Phoenix – closer to my new home.

I worked hard to build my practice once again, gaining new patients each day, and soon, the people from Iowa began to travel to me for treatments. My success with cases which baffled others and those declared incurable, brought myriads of people to my office. I worked many hard, long hours trying to keep up with the workload. And, I managed to overwork myself, and suffered a severe heart attack at the age of sixty-eight.

Regina and I again retreated to our haven in Colorado. It was a slow pull back to health, but we knew I had to give my heart a chance to gain strength. Never did consider retiring – I still had much to do. I enjoyed the cold enough and returned to Scottsdale.

Returning to practice was gradual. In 1965 I joined an old friend, Dr. Paterson in his practice on Indian School Road in Scottsdale. I worked with him for about seven months, and then moved into my own office at the Professional Plaza Building in Scottsdale.

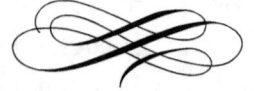

# BIRTH OF A GIANT - 8

Often the word "Miracle" comes up – but we discovered that it isn't at all appropriate. Doc insists that his treatments are plain and ordinary "Body Mechanics." He calls himself: "God's Mechanic." He offers as an explanation an analogy of an old Model T Automobile. If you are driving down the road, and your fan belt comes off – the automobile will start running rough, and overheating. If you pull into a service station with the overheating complaint – the mechanic might say: "I have a system coolant additive that will make it run much cooler." So he adds can after can of special additives – but the automobile keeps running hot and rough. You can keep trying this strategy – but the automobile won't run better until you replace the fan belt.

"Modern" medicine is much like this. You can add drugs and do surgery, but until mechanical corrections are made – nothing is going to get much better. Body Mechanics is based on the belief that God created the body of man perfectly designed, just as one would design any machine. It consists of a skeletal frame which must be in good articulation so that the muscles and ligaments can work freely and without friction, just like the pulleys and belts of any machine must be in good alignment for optimum efficiency. The organs of the human body may be compared to those machine parts. Some organs move up and down with each breath, others rock back and forth, such as the moving parts of a machine. If organs are blocked, or out of their sockets – you have problems. Restoring the order and function of the body brings back health.

"I first check the pulse on both sides of the neck. There are a dozen possible different pulses – and each defines a problem area. If I feel a strong pounding effect – I know there is an obstruction, and the heart is trying to force blood past it. If I feel a light – wispy pulse, I know that the heart sack is being pulled down – restricting the heart movement. If I feel a strong heat – pushing my hands away – I know that I am not supposed to work on this person."

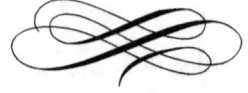

# My Awakening - 9

I'm Mike Martin, and I met Doc Huls through my Mother. She kept telling me stories about this miracle worker. I'm a Reporter in Broadcast News, and everyone tries to pull something over on us – and I didn't see anything different here. After an hour of stories in the car – I finally turned to Mom and said: "Does he walk on water also?" It got very quiet in the car, and a bit frosty for Arizona. A few weeks later, I was having some allergy problems and breathing problems. So I decided to go see this miracle. I can't accurately describe what he did, but he worked a lot on my chest and abdomen. Later – in the mirror, it looked like a football team ran across my middle with cleats on. I had a field of bruises. After a few treatments, I could breathe again. And the Allergies turned out to be toxins from some intestinal parasites. Later treatments fixed some lower back problems, and neck pains.

Doc fixed a Hiatal Hernia on Mom – where the stomach presses up against the diaphragm – with real breathing problems. I had a long and painful apology for my mom. I later discovered that the Hiatal Hernia was kind of a specialty for Doc. And he found some of his patients in an unusual way.

He treated a gentleman who spoke little English – and a lot of Italian for the Hiatal Hernia problem. About 4 months later, another gentleman who spoke a lot of Italian, and no English showed up. But he had a note – from the other gentleman – who, as it turned out, was the secretary to the Pope (several Popes ago....) He also had the Hiatal Hernia, and the note asked him to treat it. For the next 7 or 8 years, Doc ended up with the "Italian with a note" scenario 2 – 3 times a year. One patient from this country – referred by the secretary – wasn't impressed with the treatment – even though it worked. It seemed too simple. He was sure the stomach would slip out of the socket in a few weeks or months, so he bought a house in Scottsdale, and moved there with his wife. After 2 years, he finally accepted that it had worked, and sold the house.

One week, I joined a treatment in progress. Several months before, Doc received a call from Japan asking for help with a 3 year old boy. The call was from a prominent religious leader. He explained that his son was born deaf and blind – and wasn't making any progress. So a surgery was performed – and now the boy made no sound, no movements. Then 2 additional unsuccessful surgeries were done. The leader asked that Doc see his son. Doc refused.

Doc explained that he would have no way of knowing what damage had been done by the 3 surgeries. A few days later, an assistant to the leader showed up in Doc's waiting room – with the boy. He pleaded for Doc to evaluate him. Doc finally agreed – reminding them that it was unlikely he could help. He worked on the boy for half an hour a day for a week. By the end of the week – the boy was moving – and crying. That was considered a success – and the slow progress continued in Japan.

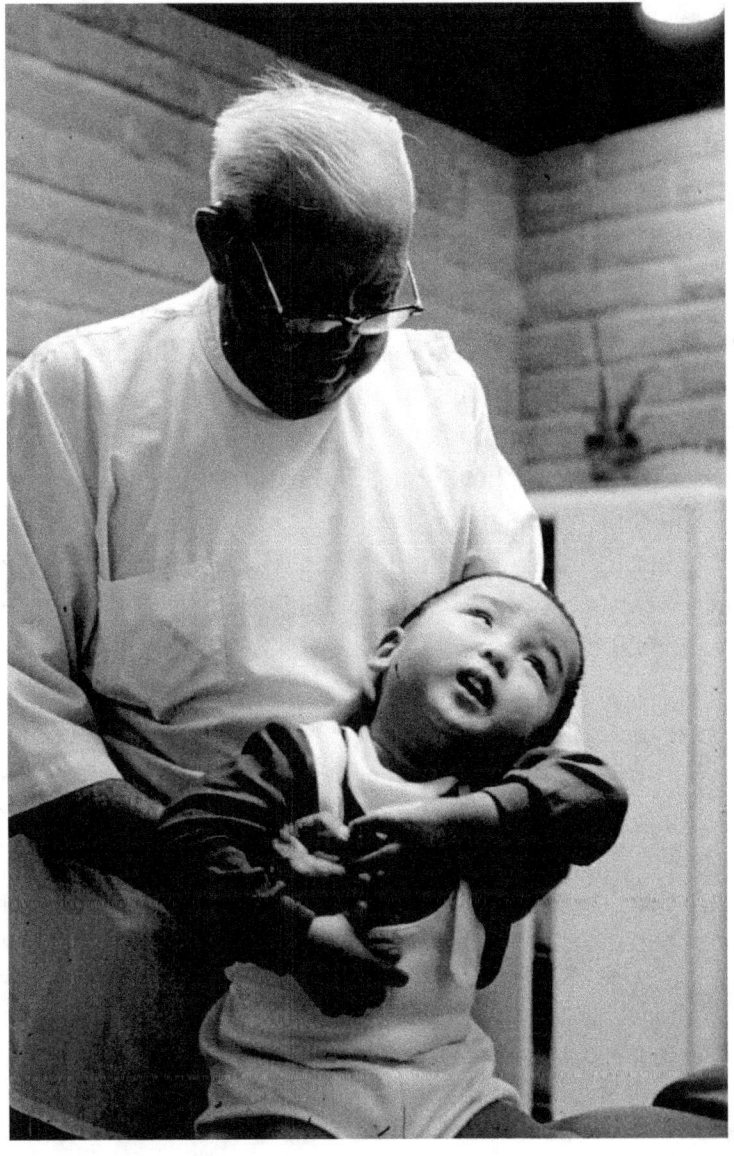

I was in the office for a return visit. Doc was checking his pulse, and the boy would stop making noises whenever Doc spoke. I realized that he now had some hearing. Then, the boy lifted his left leg – looked right at it – then reached out with his right hand – and grabbed his leg. So he was seeing shapes. I lost track of him, but heard from Betty that the boy continued making progress and was able to speak, walk, and attend school.

I wrote a news story on Doc – came out pretty well. But – due to his advanced age, we decided to film some of his work, on 8mm film – pretty much all we could afford. We hadn't tested the equipment – so when I had a chance to watch an interesting treatment – we decided to not chance the new equipment. It's my greatest regret. This was another boy – but about 12 – and a disaster. He was in a "custom wheelchair" which was actually a rolling stretcher that was bent in the areas where he couldn't. His legs were off to the right side, the right leg was 4 inches shorter than the left, and the knee cap was not attached – lying loose beside the leg bones. The arms and legs were less than 3 inches in diameter. His chest was arched up, his lower lip was curled down, and there was a noticeable ridge from the top of his head – down his forehead. His arms and legs were very thin. He was spastic on motions, and unable to Bathe, Dress, or feed himself.

The mother and father talked with Doc and mentioned that he was dropped at birth, and years later his wheelchair rolled down a hill and into a swimming pool at a corner. The boy hit the corner of the pool with his head, and sank face down to the bottom – but was quickly rescued. Doc said he could help the boy – it would take about a dozen visits – and the cost would be $400. The Mother took the boy's sister to the waiting room – the Father stayed with the boy.

OK – I have to admit that I was more than skeptical. I've seen Doc do amazing things – but this looked solidly impossible. Doc noticed that I wasn't sold on this, so he called me over, and explained things as he went along. The boy was under light anesthesia, and I could have used some also. Doc pointed to his shoes – with weights on the sides to try to balance him so maybe he could learn to walk. Doc pointed to the hips and said the weights won't do anything as long as his hips are out of the socket. With this thought, he grabbed each leg in turn – pulled it to about a flat 90 degree angle to the side – fished a bit to catch the leg bone in the hip socket – then leveraged it into the socket. The boy now had his legs lying flat and straight – not at the former awkward angle. Doc then points to the right knee, and points out that the kneecap is lying loose next to the leg bones that are overlapping. He takes both upper and lower leg bones, and hooks them into the knee cap, and straightens out the leg – which is now the same length and size as the other one.

This is beginning to get to me – as I realize what I am watching. It qualifies in my mind as a miracle – but I realize it is just Body Mechanics. Doc is putting a body back together.

Now Doc starts working on the lower abdomen. He says there is a "band" out of place – similar to a tendon – but that's not what it is. He starts digging in and working his thumbs forward very slowly from right to left near the waist – and I can see a line just below the skin – similar to the string on a bow and arrow – moving slowly in front of his thumbs – then as it reaches about the middle of his abdomen – it drops down, and the boy's chest relaxes down to the table – and the boy's breathing becomes easier.

Next – Doc points at the ridge on his forehead and states that at birth – the two halves of the skull overlap – and later expand and fuse together. He says these plates are caught. He looks me in the eye and says: "Watch carefully. His face will dance, move, expand, and contract noticeably for the next half an hour. His face will be completely different. It will continue at a much slower pace for the next month. Watch carefully – you'll never see this again in your lifetime."

Doc moved to behind the kid's head, and started massaging – and looking for something. After a couple of moments he says: "There it is." He makes a small movement at the back of the skull, and the ridge goes away – and there is a small squirt of blood that leaves his mouth, and hits the wall 10 feet away and about 8 feet up the wall. I was really feeling the need of anesthesia strongly now. The boy's head was now noticeably a bit wider – no ridge – and looked somewhat more normal.

Doc then said the jaw was out of the socket on both sides, so with one hand on each side, makes a move – and the lower lip moves up to a normal position. Then his right brow turns bright red – swells up – shifts a bit right – then sinks down to its normal position. Then the left lower jaw – then the left brow – then some chin and neck – and other larger and smaller areas. His face danced for 30 minutes.

At this point – the Mother and Daughter enter the room. She takes one quick glance at her son – then turns to Doc and says: My neck and back are bothering me from carrying my son around the house. Can you fix it?" Her husband is crying. I'm crying. Betty is crying. His sister is crying. The mother shows NO emotion and asks for help with her back and neck. I didn't need that. Doc treated her – but didn't say much.

A couple of years later – Doc said: "Mike – There's something I want to show you." He walks to a small 4 drawer chest of drawers. The first drawer is stuffed with letters. He looks for a while, and then moves to the second drawer – just as full. On the third drawer – he pulls out a letter and a photo of the kid playing baseball. His stance isn't great – but his smile is fantastic. This is the boy that couldn't bathe, clothe, or feed himself – and he is playing baseball. How much better does it get than that?

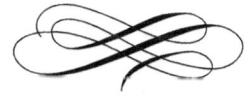

# THE OSTEOPATHIC OATH

I do hereby affirm my loyalty to the profession I am about to enter.

I will be mindful always of my great responsibility to preserve the health and the life of my patients, to retain their confidence and respect both as a physician and a friend who will guard their secrets with scrupulous honor and fidelity, to perform faithfully my professional duties, to employ only those recognized methods of treatment consistent with good judgment and with my skill and ability, keeping in mind always nature's laws and the body's inherent capacity for recovery.

I will be ever vigilant in aiding in the general welfare of the community, sustaining its laws and institution, not engaging in those practices which will in any way bring shame or discredit upon myself or my profession.

I will give no deadly drugs to any, although it be asked of me.

I will endeavor to work in accord with my colleagues in a spirit of progressive co-operation, and never by word or act cast imputations upon them or their rightful practices.

I will look with respect and esteem upon all those who have taught me my art.

To my college I will be loyal and strive always for its best interests and for the interests of the students who will come after me.

I will ever be alert to adhere to and develop the principles of osteopathy as taught by Andrew Taylor Still.

Doc had some problems – many brought on by himself. While there are several Osteopaths in Phoenix, Doc was the only Manipulative Osteopath. Most Osteopaths differ very little from your standard MD. Since Doc's methods are different than MDs and DOs – sometimes his results are much better than standard treatments. One lady received great results on a problem treated by a nearby regular Osteopath for 20 years. She asked Doc why the other DO wasn't successful. Doc – very diplomatically – answered: "Because he is an idiot and doesn't know how to do anything." She marched over to the other doctor's office and cursed him out – and quoted Doc. That happened often enough that several nearby DO's developed a bit of hatred for Doc.

So one day a Pharmacy Board investigator showed up on a regular visit and was shocked at what she found. Doc kept a LARGE Brandy Sniffer on Betty's desk in the waiting room. After treating some patients – he told them to dump their Prescription bottles into the Brandy Sniffer – they didn't need them anymore. So our investigator walked in on roughly 2 quarts of loose prescription drugs out on an open desk. It didn't go over well.

But the final straw was a travesty all around.

An ASU student and employee had a traffic accident – No Seatbelt – traveled through the passenger side of the window landing face down on the hood. A week later she was in a second accident – but this time only broke the window with her head. After some treatment – she went back to work. But it wasn't the same. She worked in a computer room – and fainted – unconscious on the floor for about 20 seconds – every day – usually twice. Then it extended to a minute – then two. When it reached 20 minutes – twice a day – she went to a neurological hospital for tests. After a week of tests, including her favorite - the famous dye in the veins – suspended upside down in a chair for hours at a time torture fest – the results were in.

**Not caused by the accidents – Genetic – incurable – here's some experimental medicine – you have no more than 6 months to live – Pay the cashier \$40,000 please.**

Over the next 2 months, 20 minutes turned into 2 hours unconscious twice a day. Finally some friends convinced her to see Doc as a last resort. They wheeled her in, Doc checked her over, told them to discontinue all medicine, and bring her back in at 6 the next morning. 12 treatments - $400. She had swelled to almost double her size, and was unconscious – carried in on a stretcher by her family and friends. Doc worked on her a little each hour all day. At closing time she was close to her normal size – walked out – Thanking Doc.

### *So what could go wrong with that?*

### *Treatment success – low cost – no problem.*

Until she turned in a $400 bill to her insurance company. They now had $40,000 paid bill that said she couldn't possibly be cured, a bill for $400 and a live patient with no after effects – back at her computer programing job at the University. When the Osteopathic Board caught wind of it – they were overjoyed! They now had a chance to eliminate their most constant thorn in the side - they filed to have a hearing to remove his license.

# LICENSING HEARING ORDERED FOR SCOTTSDALE OSTEOPATH

*"... Charges of mental impairment, ignorance or deliberate fraud endangering his patients."*

Arizona Republic, November 18, 1972

A three D.O. panel heard the case – kind of. I walked in with film camera rolling and noticed one D.O. sleeping and snoring with his head on his arms on the desk, the second D.O. was reading a newspaper held in the air, and the third D.O. was asking questions. When he spotted my camera – he knocked the paper out of the 2nd D.O.'s hands, and belted the sleeping DO hard enough to leave a bruise. The hearing continued – with a bit more professionalism.

## First question: "PROVE IT! Show us."

Local Osteopaths testified that they had not seen any before and after x-rays nor lab tests." Doc: "I don't take x-rays. They needlessly endanger the patient – and I already had all the information I needed from my examinations." They ran the hearing for a week – at hours that Doc would normally be sleeping.

The small panel controlled the hearing with an iron hand. Claims by his patients who asked to testify in his behalf were discredited because they were not experts in the medical field. Professional medical men who also asked permission to speak were discredited because of the unorthodox procedures in their own practices, due to their previous association with Dr. Huls years before. Other local Osteopaths testified that they had never witnessed Dr. Huls in practice, but felt it was impossible to do the type of manipulation and treatment he was claiming in his daily work.

In March of 1973 after a few months of appeals and various legal contortions, he was suspended from his practice for two years. During this interim he was ordered to take 100 hours of specific courses, aimed at updating his techniques. Subjects were to include:

Intracranial injuries
Diabetes mellitus
Diseases of the Prostate
Anesthesiology
Cardio-pulmonary diseases
Cardiac Resuscitation
Pharmacology and Toxicology

(None of the courses were currently available conveniently anywhere in the country.) Their findings were that Doc was way out of date. Doc was 73 years old.

The Arizona Board of Osteopathic Examiners had publicly and officially taken a stand against the principles and Oath offered by Dr. A. T. Still. They ruled against reinstating Dr. Huls on the grounds he was using archaic and outmoded techniques and was too old to continue his practice without endangering his patient's well-being.

Patients begged the board to reconsider. One father with a retarded child who had just started treatments with amazing results pleaded for permission for his son to continue his treatments. Without finishing the treatments – his son was reverting. I've never seen a man so racked with tears. And the college student/employee begged, cursed, and accused them of convicting doc on a completely successful treatment. She said: "The neurologists were wrong – completely wrong – take away **THEIR** licenses." The board got what they wanted – they got rid of a problem.

One of the hearing officers was so poisoned with hate that he died suddenly within the next year. Another retired and left the area.

Doc's attorney developed an "Out of Sight – Out of Mind" strategy and on June 13, 1974 Doc opened an office in Fountain Hills – 30 miles from his old office as a Japanese massage technique therapist. His continuing clients didn't care that he was now just a licensed Masseur. His first client was the man with the retarded son – who made a full recovery. Once the word spread of his return to practice, again patients began to return – some from half-way around the world. Every couple of months, an ugly old blue school bus would show up in the parking lot, and dozens of Mennonite people would fill the small waiting room. Their village – due to primitive medical conditions – had a problem with births and retardation rates reaching 15%. After Doc worked on the young children – the rate dropped to less than a percent.

Shortly after Doc's reopening, a medical school in Mexico offered to pay all expenses to move and relocate his family so he could teach classes in their country. It was a hard decision, but due to his age – Doc had to decline. Doc continued working 4 days a week – mostly early morning hours. He never took vacations because he said that he couldn't stand the thought of someone suffering needlessly because of his absence. He realized he had a responsibility to help his fellow man through the grace of God.

On one of his days off, he suffered a stroke, and a few weeks later on November 22, 1976 he passed away. In those few years, he was able to complete the treatments he had started, and also trained a small group in his techniques. I realized that – for me – this had been a once in a lifetime opportunity. It was much like meeting a Gandhi or Mother Theresa type of person. He was as good as it gets.

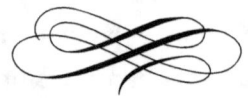

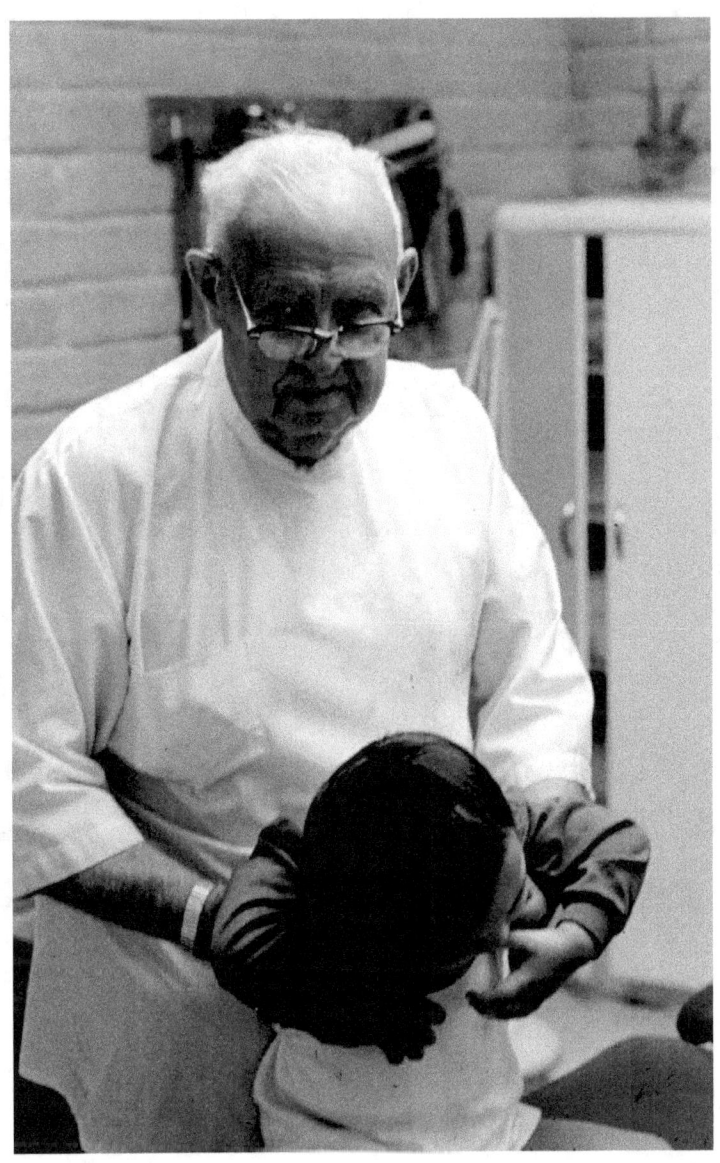

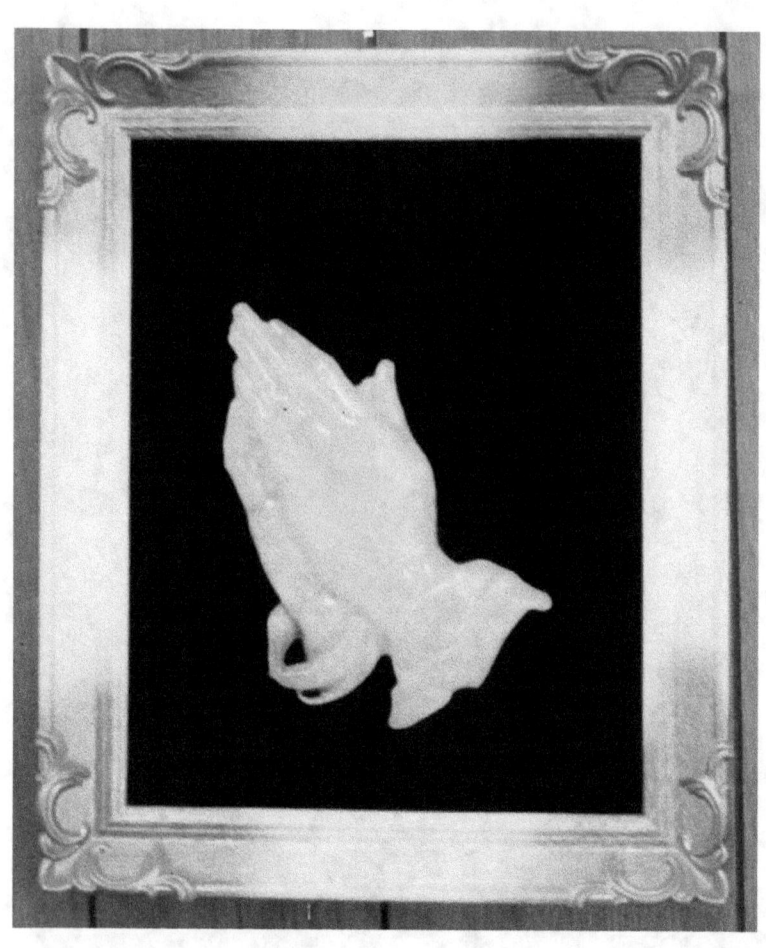

# Appendix 1 – Bits and Pieces

It was pitiful to watch him try to get out of the chair. Although he was not yet fifty, he struggled to push himself from the seat. Once standing, he grasped his two canes with desperation and began his trek to the treatment room. Back bowed, he shuffled slowly, perspiration beading his brow, the pain reflected in his eyes. The canes had been his almost constant companions for the last two years, ever since the accident. He had been everywhere - - to everyone - - and no one had been able to help him. Arthritis they had decided. Having heard of Dr. Huls from a friend, he could do no less than try.

Examination showed the cause to be skeletal displacement, not arthritis, so treatment could be given. There were straps and blocks to hold the body in such a manner that the vertebrae and muscles could be realigned into normal position. Momentary discomfort on occasion accompanied the various manipulations necessary, but soon the treatment was finished.

Gently he was helped from the table. Moistness hinted in his eyes, for he was standing erect, shoulders no longer hunched. The shadow of constant pain was absent from his face. Without his canes, he walked back and forth across the small room. His hands were reaching out instinctively for the wall if he should have need of support. Only moments after his treatment, he could sit down and get up from a chair without assistance. Relief and acceptance began to register for first there was a small grin, then a chuckle and a shake of the head. A full scale laugh echoed through the office as he bid everyone a hearty farewell a few minutes later, and left the office, the canes dangling haphazardly on his arm....

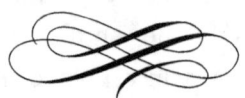

You could hear the raspy, labored breathing before you even entered the room. So tiny to be struggling for life, all of her six years had been spent fighting for a natural breath we take for granted. Coughing, gagging, sometimes unable to even utter a cry of discomfort, she had what we commonly call asthma. All the specialists had agreed on this, with a future of possible emphysema.

Examination revealed a cause, a restriction in the diaphragm area. As the mother squeezed her hand reassuringly, she felt momentary discomfort as the doctor freed the restriction. Then the tummy, which had lain so motionless during previous aspirations, rose with the next breath, expanding well past the navel. She was taking a full breath of air now, perhaps for the first time. One almost felt as though you were experiencing her very birth. Later, as she played around the room, it was explained that it would take a few days for the congestion in the lungs to clear. She would cough up much of the mucus which had collected there, due to the lack of motion, but soon she would be running and whooping just as fast and loud as the other children. The mother took the small hand in hers and began to leave the room. "Mommy," the tiny patient crooked her finger for a closer ear, "Mommy, is this what they call living?" Unable to get past the lump which was lodged in her throat, the young mother merely nodded. The little girl pulled away suddenly from her mother and ran back to the kindly doctor. Quickly throwing her arms about his neck she whispered, "thank you", kissed him, and scurried back to her mother's waiting hand and disappeared around the corner of the hall….

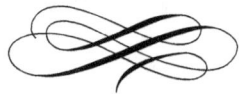

He didn't expect the doctor to be able to do anything about the tumor the specialists had found in his colon, but he was hoping for some relief from the bronchitis which had been plaguing him. Examination showed a restriction in the diaphragm area which was corrected and free breathing restored. Further examination indicated a colony of parasitic worms in the colon… After purging with the proper medication, the "tumor" was gone!

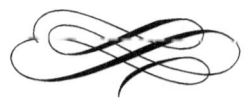

She had been sitting outside in the mall and heard some patients talking as they left his office. After 30 years as an R.N. she was going to be forced to retire early because of her legs. They just wouldn't hold her up anymore. Doctors had sadly informed her she had arthritis in her knees. Nothing they could do for her. Just take aspirin and stay off her feet as much as possible. The examination showed no arthritis, only that her knees were dislocated. Treatment left the patient able to bend her knees, stand comfortably, good balance and support and prognosis hopeful.

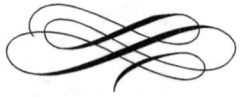

As a young man of only 35, he had a prostate problem so severe he was contemplating surgery. Examination showed that the bladder was restricted, giving the frequent urination and other symptoms. Correction of the restriction relieved all symptoms almost immediately. Surgery later proved to be unnecessary.

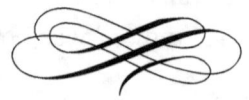

She was sixty, and there had been a lot of breast cancer in the family, but it was so painful she hoped for some relief. Examination showed only a rib displacement. Treatment and correction removed the "lumps" in the breast. Surgery again proved unnecessary....

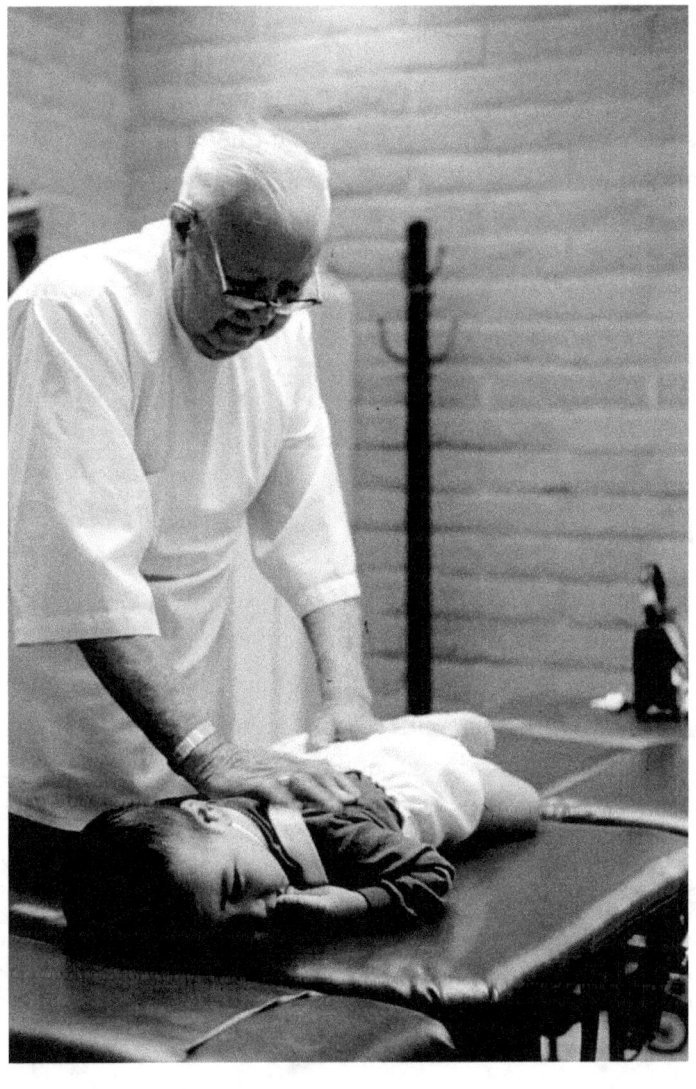

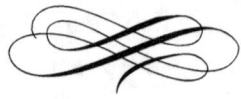

Playing soccer, the young boy had hurt his foot and was unable to walk without great pain. The x-rays had shown no fractures and specialists had said it would just take time… Examination showed several bones in the foot displaced. Treatment brought immediate relief, with walking made easy. Each day made improvement and in a few days, all symptoms were gone…

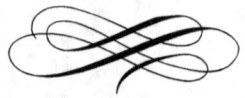

He was in his prime years, and a very good carpenter. Then he had fallen from a scaffold. Over a period of time his arms began to ache and his hand would go numb. He couldn't raise his arms above his head. He figured he had suffered a stroke or something. Doctors told him arthritis was setting in, and he should think about getting less strenuous employment. Examination showed no arthritis, only muscle displacement in the shoulders. After treatment, freedom of arm motion was immediately possible. Numbness in the hands began to lessen as the circulation was restored. Caution was given to not raise arms over the head to even put on a shirt for a few weeks, to allow the muscles to regain their elasticity.

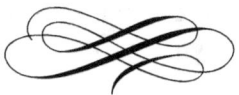

    It was quite apparent that the young lady was pregnant. This was to be her first child. She said her back hurt a lot of the time, she couldn't sit for very long in one stretch and worst of all, at 7 months, there hadn't been any fetal activity for the last few days. She had been brought in by her mother-in-law. Careful abdominal examination revealed the cause. The fetus was caught sideways in the pelvis, unable to free itself. This could be serious, even fatal for the unborn, not to mention the danger to the mother. Tilting the table with the head down at about 45 degrees angle, gentle treatment began. Moments later, freed in the pelvis, motion quickened. And tears of relief showed in the eyes of the young mother-to-be. Freeing the pelvic area, as well as releasing the fetus insured the young lady of a normal delivery. A tragedy had been averted....

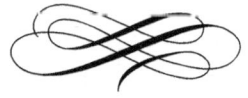

She swooped into the office like a ballerina, her laughing voice filling the room. Sighting the Doctor, her eyes sparkled and she threw open her arms and rushed to him. After a hearty kiss on the cheek, she explained she was on her way to work at the computer center, but wanted to stop and invite her "favorite boyfriend to her wedding. He accepted the invitation, and she disappeared out the door as quickly as she had appeared! Several years before, he explained, she had been brought to him diagnosed a victim of paralytic polio. Unable to walk without supports, she had been sentenced to a life as physically handicapped. As in many other such cases, the real cause was located and removed, and we had just seen the results....

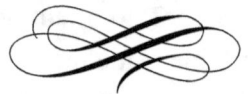

A patient returned for the 4th or 5th time complaining about terrible headaches. I felt her pulse, but couldn't find anything out of normal. I massaged her neck and spine, as I had all the times before. And I couldn't help her. I stepped out of the office to visit with an old friend – a Blind Doctor who designed and built my special treatment tables. I described my frustration at not finding the problem with my patient, and he asked to examine her. He checked her neck pulses, then ran his hand over her jaw – smiled, and said there is the problem. I ran my hand over the jaw, but couldn't spot anything. He said: "She had her wisdom teeth extracted, but one root remained in the jaw and has become infected. I thanked him, and ran my hand over the jaw a dozen more times – still couldn't find anything. She went back to her dentist – he did an x-ray – and immediately found the problem – removed the root – and no more problems.

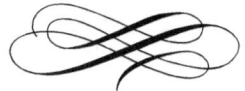

At 45 his heart was worn out, the specialists had said, and so he was awaiting a transplant when notified. He wouldn't live another six months with his own heart. His blood was so bad his whole system would soon give in, but he was resigned to the fact, he said. He had made arrangements for his family. He just came in because his friends had begged him so strongly, but he really didn't expect any "Miracles." Examination showed that both kidneys were not functioning. The laboring heart was but a symptom, not the cause. Again, there was momentary discomfort while the sensitive fingertips and hands did their well-trained job. When the treatment was over, color began to replace the ashen grey in the face. Fingertips became pink, the arms and legs became warm as if awakening from a deep sleep. As he began to move around the room he found he was not winded or as tired. A few days later a blood sample proved the clearing out of the urates (urac acid salt deposits) of the system. The surgery was cancelled, for it wasn't necessary anymore.

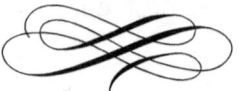

A run-away heart, the specialists called it. All she knew was that at the young age of 19 she was frail, nervous, and exhausted all the time. She had fallen off a horse a few months before, and that's when it all began. Take a lot of medication they had told her, and learn to live within her limits. Examination showed the cause. The extremely fast heart beat was the symptom; a broken tailbone was the cause. Momentary discomfort while the coccyx was reset to normal position, and in less than an hour the heart beat dropped from 200 to normal. She would need lots of rest, but in a few weeks would be able to begin to build her activities to include everything she had hoped to do with her life.

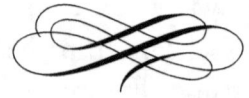

I moved to davenport because of business. I had $36,000 on the books, but couldn't collect – depression time.

Sometimes I only made 3 bucks a day. Yesterday I did 3 tonsillectomies, treated 47 people, and made $3.00. I drove out, looking for a new location. Got to Davenport, saw a man with a lunch pail (Which meant someone was working somewhere.) Saw in the paper that Davenport was one of the ten leading industrial centers in the state. I rented two rooms at a hotel, and my wife followed about 5 months later.

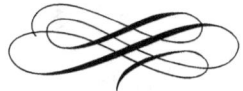

Back in 1940, at the clinic in Davenport, I never gave flu shots. I would give an injection of 2cc sterile water. When given intramuscularly, it causes antibody buildup, which protects the body naturally. I still use the same today – for boils, festering's, etc.

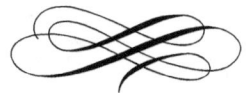

Everyone thought I would fail in Davenport. In Kirksville I had an outstanding practice. People would say "Go to the Horse Doctor" since I gave up Veterinary Medicine when I became an Osteopath. Horse Doc was used in a loving way. However, I had a patient with varicose veins. He had a sore on his leg for 17 years. A vein was feeding the ulcer on the leg. I used a solution used on horse's legs, and in 6 weeks he was healed. Ulmer Phamacal Company in Minneapolis Minnesota marketed is as VARI-CHLOR-OSE. I didn't receive any payments for it at all. Never asked and they never offered.

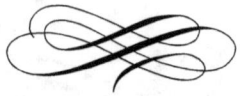

I had a boy come in, dirty as far as I was concerned with a scalp infection. He had tried for a cure, and then came to me. Long dirty hair, had to come off. We cut it down to the scalp, then kept it clean and it got well. He promised to never wear long hair again. His folks were nice people, but couldn't do anything with this boy.

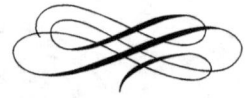

I had a 12 year old girl brought in to me, led in, she was blind. Two months later, she had 20-20 vision. Since then, she had brought in her mother, father, uncles, aunts, grandma, and others. "A child shall lead them...." She hugged and kissed me, what more could she give me? Blind by accident – Doctors said she would always be blind. Going on 3 years, and she wears no glasses.

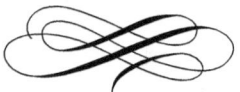

Cancer – part of the body not functioning. It lets the embryonic cells grow. I don't know. Maybe in my time I'll never know. But I bet when they do find out, it will be a malfunction of someplace. An enzyme that is not working. They're getting closer all the time. I'm lost, but if the good Lord wants me to know the answer, he will give it to me. A higher power will have to reveal it.

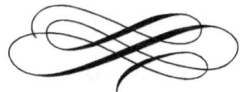

I had an incident with a drunk, found on the side of the road, after I became a Doctor. "Don't touch me, I'm dirty." I said: "Dirty on the outside, not on the inside, so come along, I'll take you home." Next day the man came to the office and swore he would not drink again. He didn't –

became the mayor and a respected man of the community. See what a kind word can do??? Never degrade anyone. Always praise and you will receive a pleasant surprise. It has a big reaction on children. Have seen a lot of people change because of a compliment.

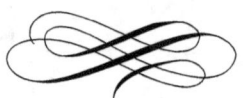

88 year old man came in on crutches. In 1927 he had been struck by lightning – dizzy ever since. In 1931 he fell and was supposed to have broken both hips and never walk again. I fixed his neck, and the dizziness left him. Went to fix his hips and he said no, couldn't fix them. I told him is dizziness had gone away, so let me try. Instead of being broken, his pubic bones (pubes) were crunched together in the front. They were overlapped and rubbed when he tried to walk. Betty and I worked together and separated those pubes, and in half an hour, he walked out carrying his canes. Betty was spell bound. This 88 year old man glowed. She said she has seen people cry, laugh, and everything, but she had never seen one glow before. To him, it was a miracle - - - to me, it was putting God's machine back together as it should be.

Isn't it strange that it stayed in, after all those years of being out? In school they told us not to treat anyone over 65, that it wasn't wise. If I hadn't treated that old man, he would still be suffering. Now he is free of pain. Sure you have to take age into consideration, and treat them accordingly. But you can still help them to better health, and save them a lot of pain they shouldn't have to suffer.

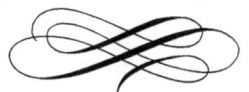

When Vitamin E became known, Dr. decided to test massive doses. The liver stopped up. Gave three dogs massive doses, two died, the third lived. Why? It turns out that his assistant had shared some coffee with the dog every morning. That dog didn't have any Vitamin E stopping up his liver. Repeated the experiment with 4 dogs, but gave two dogs coffee. They lived. What is in coffee to dissipate Vitamin E??? God gave us a natural source of a combination of manganese and caffeine. It cleans out the liver NATURALLY.

Had a Mormon patient, liver stopped up because of massive doses of E for skin condition. He could take drugs, but religion says you can't drink coffee. We got a special permission from the bishop to drink coffee if doctor is using it as a drug. Liver cleared right up.

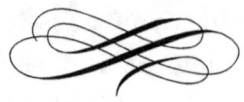

As the only son, I was trained to be a good stockman and farmer. When I was about twelve, Father sent me to town to purchase and bring back the new stock.

"Want some help over to your place?" the rancher asked, after handing me the bill of sale.

"No thank you, sir," I replied, nodding at my collie, "Vesta, my Collie, can handle it."

"Look young fella," "We know you can do a lot, but that's twenty head." Then he warned, "It's quite a piece to home and they might scatter on you."

"Thanks for your concern," I replied, "but Vesta can make it. She'll turn them without a problem." Then invited, "Come along if you just want to watch her work." "But we won't need any help."

"O.K. Vesta," I called, "let's take them home!" I signaled for her to go to the gate and handle the herd from the front, and I followed.

We had quite a crowd following us by the time we reached the fork. Vesta turned them without a blink. She knew she could look forward to an extra portion of food and attention that night!

It was a sad blow the morning I had found her, dead, her new puppies motherless. A chicken thief had ended our love affair - with poison. Life has hard facts to face, and that was one of the worst for me.

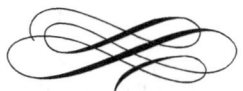

15% of Mennonite children in that community were retarded, so I was asked if I would work on them, which I did. They started bringing them in, and wanted me to work on them when they were 2 weeks old. I said I thought I could prevent it. The retardation rate dropped to less than 1%.

When the minister and his wife left, a little Jewish Doctor that had been there started talking with me. I said I wished I had a model of a perfect skull to mold those little heads after, and he said he would send me one. He sent me a picture of Christ. You wouldn't think that Jews believe that way, but this one did.

I studied that picture and got a mental picture of Christ's skull, and then I molded those baby's heads until I got a picture of this in my mind, and then I knew I was finished. I still use that method today. A baby's head will glow when I have finished. Then I know it's right. Had a little boy yesterday – His head glowed.

# Our Doctor

### By Joy Burrow

Our Dr. is the most wonderful guy.
He can fix you up from your toe to your eye.

He moves all the bones from your head to your feet.
And when he gets there you feel really neat.

I never met such a wonderful man.
There's only one like him you understand.


Tho' he's getting old now and his vision is dim,
His fingers still fly to where you are ill.

He's tried all his life to learn what he can,
About this body that God gave to man.

We all love him clearly and wish him well.
Too bad we can't help him when he has a spell.

But I guess that's the way it was meant to be.
Some folks give and others receive,

We lost him on November 22, 1976

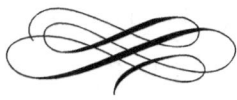

My 1<sup>st</sup> recollection of this great man was a kindly old gentleman with a twinkle in his eyes. He came in the room and said hello and asked me to sit on the table. He stood behind me and felt the pulse on both sides of my neck. He never asked why I was there or what was wrong – he first started adjusting my body. Years later I would learn what all he could do in that one treatment. Of course I didn't stop at just that one treatment. I continued to go and see him whenever I had a problem until he passed away. I am now 89 years old – still able to do housework, laundry, and cooking. I am convinced that had it not been for Dr. Huls I would not have been so lucky.

He treated several members of my family. My mother lived to be 98 – he saved her from a stroke when she was in her 80's. He treated other members of my family – my husband, son, 2 daughters, son in law, 2 granddaughters, nephew who had not been able to walk without falling. Then he learned to ride a bicycle at 6 years old.

My oldest daughter got her Aorta caught while lifting a bicycle in the trunk of her car & was dying. With one treatment it was corrected. My youngest daughter fell off a block wall when she was 3 years old and jammed her atlas up under her skull. As a result she suffered migraine headaches for 13 years until I heard of Dr. Huls. One treatment and she is now 64 years old and never has head-aches. When my son was 18 years old, he fell off a water truck and crawled into the house that night. One treatment and his back was back in place. I had a gall stone caught in the bile duct, and he moved that.

I saw so many life threatening ailments corrected in that office with simple manipulation. Just knowing what to do!!! It was marvelous to see people obtain help and health at the hands of this great man.

They came from all over the world – Japan, India, Italy, Germany, England and Mexico. He treated many Hollywood Stars – and they begged him to move to California. He said no, that they could afford to travel to Arizona. I also saw the bus loads of Mennonites and Amish who came and stayed a few days. He treated Indianapolis race car drivers. He had Doctors from Canada who came to observe and learn.

Having been a Veterinarian, he also treated our animals. You might see Greyhounds and Race horses tied up outside his office back door. I mentioned that our family dog was listless, and kept his tail between his legs. Doc asked us to bring her in, grabbed the tail, and broke a cyst – our dog made an immediate recovery.

He shared many things with me and my family from his favorite lime pie recipe to his wonderful dates and citrus.

He loved doing leather work and made beautiful belts for my Husband and Son.

The world lost a wonderful man when he died and the Osteopathic Association should forever be ashamed and embarrassed for what they did to this wonderful man and Great Doctor.

Joy Burrow

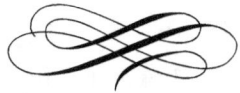

After moving a large desk at work by herself, Mom came home feeling stiffness in her back. This quickly turned into so much pain she couldn't stand up or walk. My mother was a strong woman – nothing kept her down, but she was really hurting! She quickly ended up in the hospital on traction. Five specialists saw her, and they decided she had slipped a disc and needed surgery. My brother, who had been studying with Doc at the time, begged her to go see him. With surgery being her only option, she checked herself out of the hospital, crawled into the back seat of my 4 door car, and off they went to see Doc. She crawled into his office and walked out! That was in 1973, and she had never had a recurrence – however she does still have a spot on the side of her leg that is still numb to this day.

My mother's experience was enough for our family to see how amazingly good Doc was, in fact he watched her fill out her info card and knew she had a problem with her vision. When she returned – standing on two feet, he asked her about it. Sure enough, he was right, and sure enough, he fixed it.

My brother spent two years studying with Doc, and he changed my brother for life. After Doc died – my brother opened his own office. He needed a receptionist and I need out of the medical butcher shop I felt I was working in. (Hospital) I went to work for him. Never could I have dreamed of how this was going to change my life! Just as it had been for my brother when he was studying with Doc, I witnessed more "miracles" than one could imagine. I watched a 6 year old child speak for the first time in 4 years after hitting her head on a chair! I watched formerly Deaf people cry because sounds were suddenly so loud it hurt! I watched van loads of people from out of state come to see him – celebrities, Amish from Apple Creek Ohio - It was nothing short of amazing. I couldn't get enough of what I saw.

When my brother started teaching, I was right there – And that was almost 35 years ago. I now have many of my own "miracle" stories and experiences. I have been teaching for about 15 years and this work still amazes me. I thank God, Doc, and my Brother for the incredible gift I have to help people be well. It is not me who makes them well – I am merely God's Mechanic.

Rhonda Marinakis

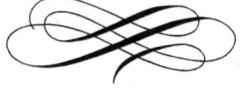

The following is a tribute to the man responsible for Myopractics. This article was printed in the Sun Valley Spur-Shopper on December 9, 1979.

*Editor's Note – Mrs. Betty Dooley, who has lived in Mesa and Tempe, has offered the following tribute to the late Dr. William J Huls of Scottsdale, who died not long ago.*

A controversial figure, Dr. Huls, before his death, encountered difficulties with state authorities because he apparently sometime adopted his own rules of procedure in treating the sick and the crippled.

Some years ago, I wrote a Zipf Code column about Dr. Huls, who had gained widespread attention because of the number of patients he was said to have helped when others failed.

There were many who swore by him and believed he could do no wrong and they remained steadfast to the very end. My attention was called to him by a number of people residing on this side of the Valley who told me of the great good he done for so many.

Mrs. Dooley is one of those. Here is her tribute to Dr. Huls:

Dear Mr. Zipf:

On November 22, the world lost a very great man, Dr. William J. Huls. At the age of 80, this wonderful man gave of himself until the day he was stricken. He was in his office at 6 a.m. every morning to help those who came

---

from all over the world for his help. It amazed me how people in Japan and other countries knew of him, yet people right here in Arizona knew very little – yet we were his chosen state.

We have five children, all very dear to us. Our first born is a very special child. When he was 18 months old, the doctors told us he would never learn to communicate with us. And it would be best for his baby brother and any other children we may have if we placed him in an institution.

We had planned from the beginning to have a large family, and no one was going to take this baby from us. We loved him and we were determined to find someone – somewhere who could help. Thus began our long search.

My husband worked overtime and began a 24 hour business to pay the ever mounting doctor bills. We took him to the finest doctors Arizona had to offer. The clinics and hospitals ran test after test. The all shook their heads and said, "Russ has hydrocephalus, and may not even live to see his seventh birthday."

It was very difficult for Russ to walk. He walked on his toes; his head was large and misshaped.

When Russ became 5 years old we enrolled him in MARC School. Only a family who has a special child can understand the joys and frustrations that took place in our lives. The love in that beautiful smile that said "Thank you" for the simple things, the things most people take for granted.

We learned so much about life from this precious gift. He loved and trusted everyone and everything. He saved little pieces of bread from his plate to share with the birds that would fly into our yard and eat right out of his hand. He could go to his grandmother's piano and play songs he had learned at Sunday school.

When Russ was 7, the doctors sat his dad and I down and said, "Look, we don't know why, but the hydrocephalus had arrested itself. The brain is damaged and can never be repaired. Russ will never go beyond the level of a 7 year old."

I asked them why he couldn't walk. They explained that the large size of his head threw his frail body off balance. That made sense and we accepted it. We took him home, loved him and began to get the best education we could to reach his limits.

He learned to ride a bicycle and swim. These were the only physical things he could do without help and he loved them.

At Washington School for the handicapped Russ received an award for swimming. His brother and sisters were so proud of him. They were always there to praise and encourage him.

In these few short years they learned more about people than most learn in a lifetime. Watching someone struggle and never give up on simple little things that come so easy for most of us.

The joys and heartaches came and went. Almost five years ago, Russ's grandmother went with a friend whose daughter is in a wheelchair to a doctor in Scottsdale.

She sat in the waiting room and saw people of all walks of life come from all over to see the very special doctor. She talked to people who flew in just for treatment. People had been in wheelchairs who could now walk – blind who could now see and those with hope that they too could be helped.

On the wall was a clipping from the Sun Valley Shopper of a story you had written about the very great doctor. Why had we never heard of him before?

Russ' grandmother told the doctor of her very special grandson and asked if he could help him. Dr. Huls smiled and said: "bring him to me and we shall see." He didn't make any promises.

She called me when she got home and said: "I'm not trying to interfere, but I made an appointment for Russell with the most amazing doctor who might be able to help him."

Russ was 11 years old then, so gentle and kind, so trusting. I felt as if God had opened a door, and if I didn't go through with it – I had failed.

The door opened and in walked the kindest, most gentle man I have ever met. I knew at that instant our prayers had been answered. He smiled and said nothing. He gently put his hand on Russ' head and reached for the information card I had filled out about Russ. Under reason for coming,

I had put "Brain damage." The doctor looked at me and asked: "Why did you say he is brain damaged?"

I replied that seven doctors had told us that he had hydrocephalus. Dr. Huls smiled and said: "This child is no more brain damaged than you or me and he's never had hydrocephalus." Sometime between birth and eight months he had an injury that you may not have even noticed at the time, but it knocked his hips out of place and forced his backbone up into the base of his brain causing pressure on the brain and forcing the skull out of shape. We are going to put the hips back in place and work the rest of his body back to the way God intended it to be. The little fellow's body has been growing crooked for almost 11 years, so we can't expect it to straighten out in a few weeks. It will take time, but by the time he is 18 years old, you will never know anything was ever wrong."

He then reached for a handmade strap and placed it across Russ' hips. Russ never said a word. He just smiled. After several minutes of work, Dr. Huls said: "Russ, get up and show mom how to walk." Russ got up and walked flat on his feet for the first-time in his life. Then the doctor said: "OK, Russ – now run around the table." And he did. All this time Russ kept saying: "Mom! Look at me, I can run." Everyone in the room was crying. I thanked God for this unbelievable man.

The next day, the school called to say Russell had kicked a football for the first time in his life. The teachers and students shared our joy. This began our uphill climb.

I began to look forward to Russ' visits to Dr. Huls. I saw miracles take place in that office. People came from everywhere. Had I not seen it for myself, I could not have believed the stories people told of how this great man touched so many lives and made so many bodies whole.

On July 2, 1972, our fifth child was born, a beautiful baby girl. Russ wanted to take her so Dr. Huls could see her. Tammie was less than a week old when Dr. Huls checked her and said she was perfect. Tammie never missed going with Russ to see Dr. Huls even at 7 a.m. She would pick him a flower and climb in the car to go see her boyfriend. She dearly loved him, and he returned her love.

About a year ago Dr. Huls had given Russ a treatment. He looked up at me and said: "Well mom there's no stopping him now. He's on his way; I've done all I can. It's up to him now."

He then had a long Man-to-Man talk with Russ. He told him to set his goals in life and never stop until he got there. "Don't ever let anyone tell you, you can't. You can do anything you set your mind to."

Dr. Huls was very proud of Russ. He helped him cope with growing 12 inches in 12 months.

Today Russ is 15 years old. He is a 6' 6.5" sophomore at Marcos de Niza High School in Tempe. He's a member of Junior Achievement. He takes classes like aviation and piano. There's no stopping him now.

We paid our last respects to Dr. Huls on November 24.  All five children stood beside him as he lay there.  No one said a word.  We lost a very special person.  It was god who had sent him to us.  Now his work was done and he was taking his long earned rest in peace.

We loved him and we shall miss him.  He gave us so much. It's up to Russ now.

Sincerely,
Betty Dooley

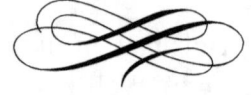

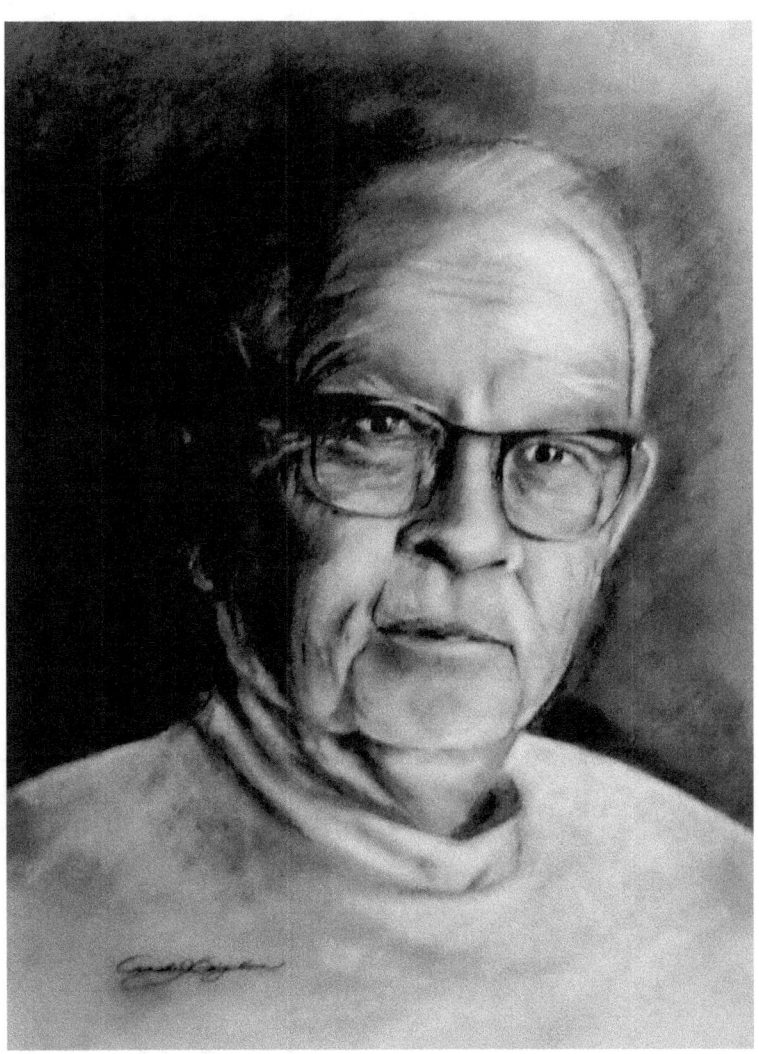

# APENDIX II – Still & Lyda

Kirksville College had an interesting history. Dr. Still was an MD at the local hospital. One winter, the town had an outbreak of Spinal Meningitis mostly among the younger people from middle school. Dr. Still worked long hours at the hospital, but there wasn't any cure – so he mostly watched the children of his friends fade away and die.

After a particularly long day, he returned home exhausted, and realized that his daughter was to be its next victim. He tried everything that had any chance of helping, but she continued to fade. The second day, he realized that his daughter wouldn't make it through the night. He was a Doctor, and he couldn't even help his own daughter.

He sat in an old wooden rocking chair, holding his daughter as he alternately cried, prayed, sang hymns, and cried some more. Sometime around midnight, he felt that he should comfort her by massaging her back, and seemed drawn to some areas more than others. After hours of comforting her – in the early morning hours, he drifted into an exhausted sleep. He was awakened near dawn by his daughter sobbing softly in his arms. She was alive, and color returned to her face. He put her to bed, and ran to the hospital, and started with his nurses and the other doctors massaging the same places he had been drawn to on his daughter. No one else died of Meningitis that day – or that week.

He researched all the possibilities that similar massage and mechanical work could do, and then started a small college teaching what he had learned. He called his new practice Osteopathy. It was about working with the soft connective tissue, and structure mechanics with a very small amount of MD type surgery. After he passed away – his school and the practitioners he trained slowly moved towards more traditional medicine and surgery – and away from massage/mechanics.

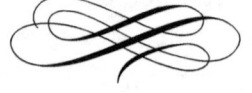

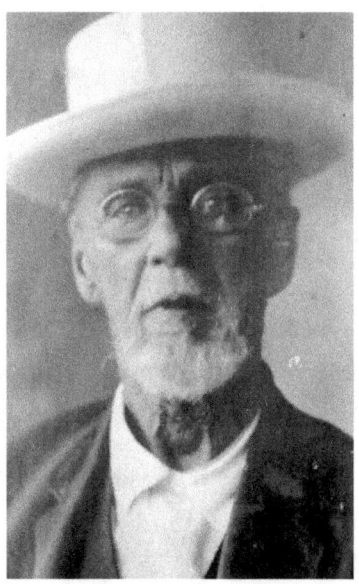

"Yes, it's been a good life" the old man said, as they walked down the road heading for the woods they both loved. He could see it was one of those days you shouldn't stay inside, with the sun blessing each leaf with its rays, and the birds singing a masterpiece in song. They walked along silently – the bird dog rushing ahead, circling and returning, just to rush off again.

Sometimes the older man would look over at the face of his young companion, waiting for a thought to take words. He loved him like a son. From the first day they had spoken to each other on a street in town, a certain special friendship had been growing between them. The young man, Roscoe Lyda had seemed attracted to him like filings to a magnet. He began following him everywhere, whenever he could. And as he grew older, he became a devoted student.  Today, as on other days, Dr. Andrew Taylor Still had something to say to his Prodigy, Roscoe Lyda.

The woods were cool and refreshing.  They made their way to their favorite spot, where the book fed into the pool the beavers had planned.  The jays squawked their protest at having been disturbed.  As the two settled down on the fallen log that several years before had become their classroom, the old dog settled near their feet for his nap.

"Yes, Roscoe, it's been hard, too," the old doctor continued, "But by the Grace of God, Osteopathy is alive and flourishing right here in Kirksville." "I was born to be a Methodist Minister, you know," the elder started out, "But I wanted into medicine.  Yep, as a young boy, 'bout the size you were when we took up together, I worked with a doctor, learning things." "Finally got some formal training," "Did a lot of doctorin' after the war broke out.  Useless slaughter, that war," he said with a frown, "no one need be a slave…" "Went into politics after that," his eyes twinkling, "had to try my hand at that, too."

"I was a general physician, treatin' those I could," he began.  "Sad to see little ones dying of fever or pox, but didn't seem to be much to help.  I've always been a religious man – raised to be a preacher.  I Carried a Bible with my medical bag.  Even now, when I need only my hands, that Good Book is close by."

"Spinal meningitis hit," he said, a frown creeping over his brow, "and everyone was losing loved ones.

Snatchin' lives up like a twister it was, here and then there... Got my family, too," he added sadly, "took them all, 'ceptin' one girl." They sat quietly for a moment, deep in their own thoughts.

"In desperation," he continued, "I took her on my lap. Her body was aching' bad. Her color and breathing was getting worse by the very minute." With his hands moving across his legs, as if reliving that time, he went on. "I closed my eyes and prayed to the Good Father to spare this child. Show me how to save her..." He sat motionless for a moment, then started again, "Well you know, Roscoe, we Osteopaths don't like to use the word rub, but back then that's all you could have called it. I rubbed her neck, shoulders, back, hips. Pushing, pulling gently, trying to bring that little body back from the grave that had called up so many others.." Shaking his greying head, he stood up, turning to face the young man.

"She lived," he said triumphantly, "and I felt God had shown me a way to save her and thousands of others. I worked like a crazy man, 'till I proved to myself that what I did for her could be done for others." His eyes misted over, just talking about it. This was the reason for his dedication through these hard years.

"It was a miracle, my daughter livin'," he declared, "but it was the miracle of Nature, of God. It was a healing that lead me to studying God's real Plan for us." He turned, looking up at the trees that made up their lecture hall, trying to ease the past from his shoulders.

"See that tree yonder?" he asked, motioning to one a few yards away. Roscoe Nodded.

"See up near the top, that scrawny limb, off to the left?"

"Yes sir, I see it." Reassured Roscoe, watching the limb.

"As an Osteopath, always keep in your mind this one thing. When you see a person with a bad spot, it's going to be like that tree. Underneath the ground, hidden, is a damaged or restricted root. "That," he emphasized, "is the <u>cause</u> of what you see up there." He pointed from the ground to the trunk and up to the limb.

"You could get up there and bandage that limb 'til you were green as a leaf, and it wouldn't do a hair of good." He warned, "Get down into that root, that cause. Free it from rocks or whatever. When that path is clear of interference and that root is free to spread, that limb will take to leafin' out and be as healthy as the rest." He turned again to face this young man that he knew was going to carry on that philosophy, and added, "Be dedicated. Help people grow the way God Planned for them to. We're all his creations, entitled to our full growth."

"You won't have all the trouble I did," Doc Still continued, sitting back down on the leg. "When I was trying to prove all this to others, I had to battle all the pressure of the community." He laughed, throwing his head back, thinking of the times he had kept people from dying, and even the preachers had called him a "devil-man."

"Called me every name in the book," he grinned at Roscoe, "and a few that still haven't been entered."

Turning more serious, he continued, "The other doctors refused to listen to me, even with all the proof I had. Years of studying bodies of Indians out there on the reservation… Checkin' that Plan God had when he created us in his image… What was normal, what happened when a certain set of bones or muscles or organs were shifted." Shaking his head again, he stated firmly, "Lots of work, and heartbreak, sometimes.. But I knew it was a good theory, a sound one."

"As I helped more people, the shouts got louder, too. Took to treating people at night, so's nobody would criticize me or them for using me." Thinking of when he was expelled by his fellow physicians, alone and without any encouragement, he added, "Those were not very happy days."

"Only one thing kept me going, Roscoe. Trust in the Lord. Faith in what I had seen with my own eyes, and proven with my own hands."

Looking at his hands, turning them over slowly, he changed the subject. "Did I ever tell you about that doctor that came to prove me a quack?"

"You've told mc about some, but which one is this?"

"This was before the school got started. I'd tried to teach a few, but they lacked the anatomy trainin to be good Operators." He shifted a little on the log to get more comfortable.

"Anyhow, one day a doctor from Scotland, across the waters, came to my door. He said he'd heard of me, and wanted to know just what the devil I was doing to people!" He chuckled, "Well, he was an open-minded fellow, which is hard to find, so after he saw a few cases and listened to the theories, he decided to stay a few days longer." He broke into a broad grin, adding, "He taught a four month anatomy class for us before he went his way." They both laughed, seeing the truth in what had happened.

"God had a hand in keeping things going, all right. Like the family name of Hamilton that called for me. The mother was ailin', and no one could seem to ease her." His kind eyes reflected his memories clearly as he continued. "Straightened her, and one of the boys, DeWitt, took to showin' their appreciation. We opened that two room school," he motioned toward town, "back in 1882; because he got us the Charter, bless 'em!"

"Handful of students, including my own boys," he reminisced, "but it took to growing, and now we're turning them out pretty good, aren't we, Doctor?" He emphasized the title, knowing how important it was to Roscoe.

Beaming, Roscoe teased back, "Thank you, Doctor." Then in a more serious tone, he asked, "Why do you think people criticize something and try to destroy it?"

Even today people are scoffing our methods of treatment, when they can see the proof with their own eyes."

"All through life," Dr. Still began, "You're going to find those who live in a world they have built for themselves.. Sometimes good, sometimes bad. Someone comes along with something that will change the shape, color and texture of that, and, well," he said, "people don't like having their world shook around."

"Osteopathy is turning the world of medicine topsy-turvy, son." Some are afraid of losin' their positions. Osteopathy is takin' the power out of the surgeons' knife and the pill, and givin' it back to its rightful owner, God."

"Someday," he continued, choosing his words carefully. "Doctorin's going to be a big business. Back in 1874, when I first declared Osteopathy a practicing science, I guess I shook a few major stockholders." He laughed with Roscoe, who seemed to catch the jest right off.

"Nobody said it would be easy," he said. "This trying to prove Osteopathy. I didn't expect it to be. Remember, Roscoe," he reminded. "Any knowledge you want, you must work for. Prove you deserve it." He gestured in emphasis. "I want the world to know about Osteopathy and what it can do for humanity. I've worked hard, and it's been worth it. It can be expanded, enlarged upon, proven further…. That's your job, now." He studied the young man alongside him… He saw strength in his face and hands, and he knew all would be well.

"I understand why the doctors are reluctant to try something so different, but why are people so slow to see its potential?"

"It seems too simple," he replied. "They'd like to accept it, but with all the sickness and heartbreak around," he defended, "It's sort of hard to see our Good Father in the right light, you see. People feel like god's forsaken them, but the Bible holds the real answer. In Isaiah fifty-nine, verses one and two, it says;

**"Behold, the Lord's hand is not shortened, that it cannot save; neither his ear heavy, that it cannot hear; But your iniquities have separated between you and your God, and your sins have hid his face from you, that he will not hear."**

"Son, use your Bible for your guide. With God, all things are possible. God created your body to function perfectly, like a machine." He leaned over to scratch the head of the dog resting at his feet, continuing, "We're made with pulleys, levers, gears, pistons, and the like, just like any other machine. As an Osteopath," he added simply, "you are God's Mechanic." He waited for roscoe's nod, and then continued. "You have studied anatomy, histology, physiology, and pathology. Your studies have included learning the true anatomical structure as God planned it."

"You must know the normal," he explained, "before you can recognize the abnormal.. do you see?" He knew he did, for this was stressed in all the classes, and he himself told Roscoe this many times before.

"When you repair the structural frame," he continued, "you are freeing God's machine to acknowledge the Great Creator of it." With deep sincerity and a tone of urgency, he persisted," Have a patient leave with more than they came in with. More health, more faith. Help those that seek, and try to understand those who are afraid of Truth. You can't change the world, so don't try. Help the body, God will do the rest."

Roscoe looked puzzled, "What do you mean, Doc?

"A little of you should go out with each patient," he began, "Let me give you an example. Suppose a parent brings in a child, paralyzed, Can't walk a lick. I treat him; he walks out, shaky of course, but recovering." He watched for a reaction, and then continued, "What would he have been without help? What," he challenged, "will he do now, with his life, with his legs restored to him?" He rested his point with silence.

"Yes, I see," Roscoe offered thoughtfully, "that we have a hand in shaping a persons' future. Like is said, "we pass this way but once..." his voice trailed off. They sat quietly, each thinking of what had just been said.

Doc knew it was soon time for Roscoe to leave. He was going to Seattle, Washington, to begin his own practice. Doc wanted him to go well prepared, but now the time seemed so short.

"You realize the importance of this knowledge. Osteopathy is a natural science. Given a chance, mans' body can fight off anything. God made us that way. He didn't take that gift of health away, we have stopped accepting it."

"In its purity," he stressed, "Osteopathy can revolutionize the healing arts."

Searching the young face, "Keep it alive, Roscoe Lyda," he said, tears filling his aging eyes.

"Don't let anyone, or anything, bury it between the lines of the page of a text book. When you find a man," he continued, "willing to serve as an Osteopath, make him work for the knowledge. Help them to be true Osteopaths. Years will change the schools," he added, "for change is constant, and we can't stop that. I've worked hard to bring Osteopathy to the light," he said, "but I'm getting older, and won't be here to protect the teachings." He sighed deeply, and then placing his worn hand on Roscoe's wide shoulder, said, "God grant man the open mind to grow and free themselves to whole bodies and Higher Knowledge…"

Their eyes met in understanding. They rose and started back to town, the dog again leading the way. It had been a good afternoon. An afternoon to remember….

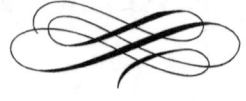

# Wedge of Time & Theory

Osteopathy, as Dr. Still perfected and practiced it, was laid to rest with his bones in 1917. Only a handful of dedicated, thinking men continued to seek after what he had first tapped. This loss of a theory and technique, perhaps considered fanatic and crude by todays sophisticated society, seems to have been a deep loss to humanity.

As he proved it, Osteopathy was based on the perfection of Nature's work. When all the parts of the human body are in line, we have health. When they are not, the effect is disease. When the parts are readjusted, disease gives way to health. The work of the osteopath is to adjust the body from abnormal to normal, and health is the result.

Dr. Still once said, "The body has its own chemical laboratory, and man can't improve on it. Disease is the effect only, and positive proof that somewhere in that machine a belt is off, A journal bent, or a cog broken or caught."

Man's power to cure is as good as his knowledge of the normal position, and his skill to adjust the bones, muscles and ligaments and give freedom to the nerves, blood, secretions and excretions. Dr. Still wholly gave credit to God for the Wisdom and skill to build a perfect machine to house the Soul of Man. Even by today's standards of spiritual understanding, this theory should hold true.

The first school or Osteopathy still stands in Kirksville, Missouri. Alongside are the modern buildings sprawled about, indicating the growth pattern. There were seven students in that first class, including Dr. Still's own boys. They went into the world to practice, without licenses, and with no legal protection whatsoever. There were no laws to help them, no precedents to follow. All they had was the strong belief and faith that they had learned something which was needed and would be helpful in easing the maladies of their fellow man.

Sometime, in that early, fragile beginning, some students lacked the anatomical knowledge of structure so important, and when their treatments failed to bring the expected results, their faith in Osteopathy waivered. They then sought, in their own frustration, to add to the Science that which they felt would be of benefit. Each class being taught by the former, apparently sped up the decline of the true Osteopathic Theory.

Change is constant. But in that change is always hidden the pitfall of decisions. Deciding what should remain, and what must fall by the wayside. All through history it has been so. We look to the future and take from the past those things with which we can mold our new way. And we can only take with us those things we can comprehend. Each generation which follows seems to only be aware of what is handed to them. Therefore, it is a simple matter to see the massive changes which have come about.

Besides the school at Kirksville, there are many throughout the land. And each year brings into society more new, young, Osteopaths. They are now protected by the Government, just as other branches of Science; they are licensed in all States, and although there is still some stigma to the position, for the most part, Osteopaths are an accepted part of our society.

However, the etiology of the Science, held so dear by Dr. Still, has been diluted by other practices and theories. Dr. Still often had reminded his students: "A coon can't climb two trees at the same time…" Meaning that you cannot take on two subjects at the same time and do either one justice. This seems to have created the problem we have today. One tree had to be abandoned, and it seems to have been the tallest and strongest one.

Today's Osteopathic schools teach the use of medications, a great deal of surgery, and the methods of diagnosis vary greatly. The investigation and study of God's Plan for Man is being left, for the most part, to the Theologians.

Let us look into Great Literature concerning man and the Bible. Tennyson makes over 400 references to passages in the Bible. Browning makes over 600. In Shakespeare, there are 700 such references. In Milton's work, they run into the thousands. Perhaps it is not just a question of dogma, theology, or religion. Knowledge of the Bible seems to be a requirement of General Intelligence.

In the book,

'THE PRACTICE OF OSTEOPATHY',

a 1920 edition, is a statement:

"Osteopathy is not as much a question of books, as it is of intelligence. A successful Osteopath is, in all cases, or should be, a person of individuality, with a mechanical eye behind all motions or efforts to readjust any part of the body to its original normality. Because unguided force is dangerous, often doing harm and failing to give relief, this should be the reward of well-directed skill."

Success, then would seem to hinge on knowing normal motion and structure. The incomplete, unguided manipulative treatments failing to reach the cause and the disease continues. And how like us to feel the technique is lacking foundation, rather than to accept the ego crushing possibility that we are lacking in knowledge of technique.

The earlier, "well-trained" technicians stood firm on his knowledge of structure of the human body, and knew thoroughness would bring results and relief. There was no doubt in his mind. And if relief was not complete, he did not hesitate, but reasoned that his adjustment had not reached the cause, and he continued to work until he located and corrected the abnormality. The words of Sir William Drummond seem appropriate here:

"He who will not reason is a bigot;
He who cannot, is a fool;
And he who dares not, is a slave."

A century has rolled past since Dr. Still declared his war on disease. Even by the 1920's, his techniques had lost credulance.  Manipulation had begun to be put into a meager position, with limited spectrum.  Physicians, who were fortunate (?) enough to receive training abroad, came back with many new methods of diagnosis, new methods and reasons for surgery, and new drugs to administer.

Specialization became the big thing, and soon sight of the body as a working unit became obscured. Remember Dr. Still's remark about the tree in the forest? The withered branch was the effect. The cause actually lay beneath the surface. Reason tells us the body cannot be dissected into "special, separate divisions."

The crucial point in today's approach to Osteopathy, or to any of the healing arts, for that matter, is as Dr. Still punctuated all his teachings. The operator must know the normal before he can diagnose the abnormal. What do we find taught in the medical schools today? In dissection and autopsies, what do they watch for, and what do they base their findings on?

Dr. Still, through his dissection studies, founded this statement:

"The power of the artery must be absolute, universal, and unobstructed, or disease will result. The moment of its disturbance mans the period when disease begins to sow the seeds of destruction in the human body. And in no case can it be done without a broken or suspended current of arterial blood."

He followed with the discovery of the <u>cause</u> of this interrupted flow of the blood stream, the theory of obstruction by anatomical displacement. And it is the only theory of the etiology of all science which seems able to stand the test of science itself, and its acceptance and practice will mean a complete change in the field of Therapeutics.

The very science of Osteopathy, as defined in the 1920 edition we quoted earlier, reads as follows:

"That science or any system of healing which emphasizes;

A – The diagnosis of disease by <u>physical</u> methods, with the view of discovering not the systems, but the <u>causes</u> of disease, with connection with displacements of tissue, obstruction of the fluids, and interference with the forces of the organism.

B – Treatment of disease by <u>scientific manipulation</u> to connection with which the operating physician mechanically uses and spplies the inherent resources of the organism to overcome diseases and establish health. This done by either removing or <u>correcting mechanical</u>

disorders, thus allowing nature to recuperate the diseased part, or by producing and establishing anti-toxic and antiseptic conditions to counteract the toxic and septic conditions of the organism or its parts.

C – The application of mechanical and operative surgery in setting fractures or dislocated bones, repairing lacerations and removing abnormal tissue elements when these become dangerous to organic life."

This publication carried much of Dr. Still's Original theories, and underlined are specific phrases which point to a well-knowledged approach to treatment, which through individual interpretation, seemed to have been overlooked, and set aside for the next publication. Then incorrect diagnosis undermined any well intended treatment which followed. Dr. Still had warned, "…do not let the truth be hidden in the pages of a book, but keep them alive…" Apparently his words were lost in the clamor…

There is a great division in the medical practices of today. Each declaring it has the answer to our woes. If, as Dr. Still proposed, the body has all the chemicals and substances necessary to maintain itself, then isn't it probable that each field of Therapeutics, no matter how trivial or absurd its system, should report its 'cures'? I would suggest that this natural law has saved more physicians from close spots than they are generally willing to admit!

But the truth behind a system of treatment should be consistent. There should be an established method of procedure, from the point of diagnosis to the final result, which should be good health. This is not true of any system applying drugs as its principle therapy.

There is no doubt that the pharmaceutical records will show drugs whose action is rapid and effective as far as securing activity or decrease of secretions. But the element of danger or destruction may be great. Often times their powers do not stop at the desired effect, or give an added, negative side effect. Each of us has probably experienced this. The use of drugs is, at best an educated guess, when it comes to the individual's reaction to them. The fact that a particular preparation helped Joe Blow, has little to do with its effect on me. Dr. Still disliked the use of drugs for that very reason.

From observation of Dr. Huls' practice, it seems True Osteopathy has a set of principles for application that are constant, consistent, and reliable. The same force that overcomes one malady will overcome others, if set into motion. Forces that produce a diseased condition will, if normalized, restore the established type. There is no need for drugs, no excuses need be given, no apologies stammered.

Any system of Therapeutics which lacks this type of constancy should investigate its premise and revise and replace its methods of treatment with those that breed constructive and health-giving results. Change in the technique and theory would not come easy, but considering the stakes involved - - humanity's health and well-being - - is there any alternative?

Did Dr. Still possess a special 'feel', or 'touch' which others cannot attain? No. He was undoubtedly a very spiritual, devout man, but his anatomical knowledge was gained from hard study.

The dissection of cadavers, with a keen eye for mechanical structure, led him to his discoveries. Cannot the medical student of today gain that same knowledge and study? Especially with modern aids such as good lighting, the microscope, and electronic technology?

Dr. Still did have a deep and extensive knowledge of the Bible, God, and Nature. But cannot the young physician of today have the same depth of understanding and awareness? In truth, shouldn't each man seek his own level or God Presence, and when found, incorporate it into his daily life? Any physician worth his single will admit that Nature heals, and rebuilds, not man! To claim a cure without Devine intervention is pure folly!

True (original) Osteopathy gives credit to God, Nature, and Universal Energy. For bringing the body back to good health. True Osteopathy claims no cures, only that it can remove the blocks from the path, so health can be restored.

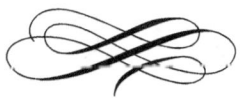

**Additional copies of this book may be purchased from:**

createspace.com

amazon.com

For information on Myopractics:

www.myopractor.com

Natural Therapeutics Inc. - 480-655-8888

If you would like more information about God's Mechanics – search for the name Andrew Taylor Still on amazon.com

All of his 4 books are back in print, including a text book. A 5th book is about a visit to his office and home at the turn of the century.

www.ingramcontent.com/pod-product-compliance
Lightning Source LLC
Chambersburg PA
CBHW060358290526
45791CB00002B/558

# Many say Dr. Huls was a Miracle Worker
# He said he was God's Mechanic.

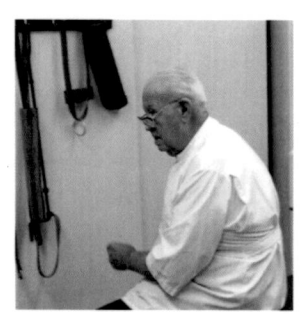

"Modern" medicine adds drugs and surgery, but until mechanical correction are made – nothing is going to get much better. Body Mechanics is based on the belief that God created the body of man perfectly designed, just as one would design any machine. It consists of a skeletal frame which must be in good articulation so that the muscles and ligaments can work freely and without friction, just like the pulleys and belts of any machine must be in good alignment for optimum efficiency. The organs of the human body may be compared to those machine parts. Some organs move up and down with each breath, others rock back and forth, such as the moving parts of a machine. If organs are blocked, or out of their sockets – you have problems. Restoring the order and function of the body brings back health.

ISBN 9781495479069

90000

9 781495 479069